NURSERY NURSING

To Nick, Belinda, St John, Justin and Anna, also all my former students, without whom this book would not have been written.

Nursery Nursing

JANET CORNWELL-MENZIES
BA, AdvDipEd, CertEd, NNEB
Principal
Hawley Place School
Camberley
(Formerly Senior Lecturer in Education
Croydon College, London)

BLACKWELL
SCIENTIFIC PUBLICATIONS
OXFORD LONDON EDINBURGH
BOSTON PALO ALTO MELBOURNE

© 1984 by
Blackwell Scientific Publications
Editorial offices:
Osney Mead, Oxford, OX2 0EL
8 John Street, London, WC1N 2ES
9 Forrest Road, Edinburgh, EH1 2QH
52 Beacon Street, Boston
  Massachusetts 02108, USA
706 Cowper Street, Palo Alto
  California 94301, USA
99 Barry Street, Carlton
  Victoria 3053, Australia

First published 1984

Set by DMB (Typesetting)
Oxford
Printed and bound by
Redwood Burn Ltd,
Trowbridge

DISTRIBUTORS

USA
  Blackwell Mosby Book Distributors
  11830 Westline Industrial Drive
  St Louis, Missouri 63141

Canada
  Blackwell Mosby Book Distributors
  120 Melford Drive, Scarborough
  Ontario M1B 2X4

Australia
  Blackwell Scientific Book Distributors
  31 Advantage Road, Highett
  Victoria 3190

British Library
Cataloguing in Publication Data
Cornwell-Menzies, Janet
  Nursery Nursing
  1. Children—Care and hygiene
  2. Day care centers
  I. Title
  613'.0432   RJ45

ISBN 0-632-00873-3

Contents

Preface

This book is written for nursery nurse students, covering the syllabus for the National Nursery Examination Board. Students who are following related courses of study in child care or development will also find that this text supports their syllabus. Although reference may be found to a comprehensive range of subjects, there is still, however, no substitute for wide reading practice. I hope that the student will be sufficiently motivated by the areas included in the book to explore in more depth those of specific interest to her.

The content is particularly aimed towards a redress of the traditional bias towards the medical aspect of the course in previous books to more emphasis on the normal development of the child, together with recommended practice which encourages such development.

Although the qualified NNEB person is known as a *nursery nurse*, the similarity between her and a Registered General or Enrolled Nurse is tenuous. One directs her skills towards preventive measures to assist positive health and normal development, the other's skills lean towards the curative. Unfortunately, some children do not develop according to the accepted normal pattern. This deviation may be found in any single area, such as deafness, or in a combination of two or even more. Whether these children are cared for with others displaying similar problems, or integrated into a school or nursery whose groups or classes do not present such needs, nursery nurses will have a distinct role. Likewise, in the hospital setting, long or short stay patients will be emotionally, socially and intellectually supported by the nursery nurse. She, through her training and experience, will be sensitive to the influence which physical illness may have on the other aspects of growth and development.

Normal human development is covered up to the eighth year, together with some of the special needs which may be presented during this period. As well as textbook advice, there is frequent reference to the realities of caring for young children. The section entitled 'Observing Children' (Chapter 12) supports this important element within the examination syllabus. Throughout the book, reference to the value of observation is emphasised where relevant.

Nursery nurses have a range of opportunities available to them after qualification. Some of these are looked at in Chapter 13. It is not possible during the two year course to offer experience in all the employment areas, but the student should be aware of them. This section aims to give an informative overview. Appendix 1 presents the very extensive range of skills which may be expected of the nursery nurse. It reflects the considerable demands of the course and the attention given to areas often not appreciated.

I hope that the reader already considering a career with young children will be convinced of the value of such work, and that she will throughout her life be able to draw upon the knowledge, attitudes and skills, discovered, acquired and developed during her training.

One of the most important aspects must be, that learning is never complete, there is always something new and exciting to discover.

Acknowledgements

I would like to thank Margaret Bonham for patiently typing much of the manuscript and my husband for typing the rest, and helping with reading of the proof. To Blackwell Scientific Publications and Phyllis Holbrook, the editor, my thanks for their encouragement to write this book, with especial thanks to Griselda Campbell for seeing the work through from manuscript to bound book. I also thank Leslie Fahidy for some of his photographs, and the Netherne Hospital Day Nursery and the Weir Day Nursery for their photographs. Finally, my thanks go to my family for their patience and support.

Chapter 1
Overview of Development

Happily, most children grow towards maturity with relatively few problems being displayed. It is easy to assess when a child's physical development is progressing favourably, and with little study, we can become skilled at identifying that which is outside the 'normal' range. Social development is also observable, and this behaviour once again is easily assessable. Intellectual and emotional development are more complicated. They are difficult to assess or measure, and no-one has yet presented the world with a universal model for such measurement.

DEVELOPMENTAL STAGES

To uncover the mysteries of these hidden areas of human development, various theorists (Piaget, Freud, Lewin, Skinner, Gesell) have presented their ideas.

JEAN PIAGET

Jean Piaget, born in Switzerland, was for over 50 years involved in the study of children's intellectual and moral reasoning. He began as a biologist, and went on to practise as a psychologist, using his own children as models for observation purposes. Clearly this does set its own limitations. Piaget proposed that all children passed through a series of stages, that these stages never varied in order, but that one may overlap the other. He concentrated on the normal, average child.

The *sensory-motor stage, 0-2 years*, is when the child's relationship with his or her environment is organized and experienced through the senses. This starts with accidental learning resulting from the basic exploratory drive, together with conscious efforts made by the adults in his or her world.

1

The *preoperational stage, 2-6 years,* begins with a period of egocentrism, when the world is seen solely through the eyes of the child, and from his or her point of view. Reasoning is fairly primitive, and conclusive. Between the ages of 3 and 5 years it has been shown that some children are already moving out of this stage. At 5 or 6 years the concept of reversibility may also emerge, and the solving of problems can be organized by forward and 'backward' thought.

The chronological boundaries are more flexible within the *concrete operations phase, 6-12 years.* The beginning of this period is illustrated by the child's ability to manipulate conceptually, i.e. to organize numbers, by adding, subtracting and sharing; by grouping objects logically and arranging them in order. All such actions need to be related to actual practical experience. During this period such skills continue to develop and improve, consolidating over the next 5 or 6 years.

The *formal operations stage* emerges once the preceding stage is negotiated satisfactorily, the age not necessarily identifiable. All adults, however, may not reach this developmental level, sufficiently prepared to achieve further skills. The stage is illustrated by the ability to imagine and organize, and to search logically and systematically for solutions to problems. They do not normally resort to trial and error, or random guesswork.

SIGMUND FREUD

Sigmund Freud's theories were based on the childhood recollections of patients treated for neuroses in his psychiatric centre in Vienna. Note the caution one would need to apply therefore in drawing generalities from these specifics. He agreed with Piaget's theory of stages, but concentrated on psychosexual development. In this way he follows personality growth through ways in which children's sexual drives are satisfied from one stage to another.

KURT LEWIN

Kurt Lewin uses the term *life space* as the combined forces which influence the child's behaviour at any point. The forces he identifies are: *physical,* including the immediate environment as well as the person; *emotional,* and *mental,* including the set of memories and experiences, which influence any action. Obviously this 'set' changes from day to day, even hour to hour, as a human builds on experience and adds fresh information, in either an active or passive manner. In decision-making, the stronger forces determine the outcome.

Lewin probably pays more attention to adolescence than most of the other theorists. He sees the period as one of puzzlement for the young person, and compares it to a journey through strange territory, without the aid of an efficient map or guide. He also suggests that adolescent behaviour may be as difficult to understand, and come to terms with, for the person experiencing the period, as for the spectator.

B. F. SKINNER

B. F. Skinner, an American psychologist, prefers to observe the influences which may determine a certain behaviour, rather than try to interpret what may be the pattern of thought behind the action. This view is termed *behaviourism.* Skinner presents the theory that if the consequences of an action are pleasant, the behaviour will be repeated. If the consequences are unpleasant or painful, the reverse will be the case. Therefore behaviour patterns are established according to previous experiences. Obviously some examples would confirm this view without much argument. If, whenever you had struck a match, the flame had burned your fingers, the action of striking a match would be made either under extreme pressure or after taking elaborate precautions. Think about Skinner's theory in relation to discipline for young children. Follow these thoughts through to adolescence, and consider some of the possible problems.

ARNOLD GESELL

Arnold Gesell was another American exponent of human development. He agreed with Piaget and Freud, that all children pass through similar stages and accompanying identifiable common behaviour, but he presented that the force behind the pattern is based within the inherited genetic code. This may be referred to as the *biological clock*. The term *maturation* was originally Gesell's, and he refers to the unfolding of an established plan as the cause of an inviolable pattern of development. In other words, that everything is stored until the appropriate moment for its unwrapping—a set of developmental time capsules.

Summary

A very brief summary of some of the ideas presented reflects four of the most well known theories.

1 Piaget, as the *cognitive theorist*. This theory emphasizes the development of thought processes.

2 Freud, as the *psychoanalytic theorist*. This theory concentrates on the development of personality.

3 Skinner, as the *learning theorist*. This theory focusses on how learning takes place, but argues with the sequential idea presented by both Piaget and Freud.

4 Gesell, as the *maturational theorist*. This theory is based on biological arguments for the emerging pattern of development of all human beings.

General overview

In the study of child development, and in the area of practical child care, there are fewer 'rights' and 'wrongs' than there are real alternatives. The many theoretical views all have some credence, and some will appeal to the individual more than others. Sometimes, elements of more than one will be accepted into a total viewpoint.

Obviously in areas such as safety and first aid there are sharper lines defining right and wrong, but even in first aid treatment what was considered correct practice years ago may no longer be recommended. For example, the treatment of shock, burns and drowning have all changed within the last 20 years or so. The Falklands Crisis (1982) stimulated an effective, pioneering approach to the emergency treatment for burns, that of irrigation with a solution containing a chlorine-type base, followed by the exclusion of air, in plastic bags where appropriate.

Many approaches to discipline will be expressed by parents and child care practitioners. It is impossible to agree with all of them. What is most important is, having carefully and intelligently identified the needs of children, their variation, as well as common areas, you seek to meet those needs effectively and harmoniously. Accept that the views of others may well have something of value to offer, but never be afraid to express doubts whenever a particular practice gives rise to reasonable concern. Your first duty is to the children in your care. It is misguided loyalty to ignore such observations as unreasonable persuasion to eat, to sleep, or to overcome natural or acquired fears. Discuss these experiences with the tutors at College. There may often be a logical explanation. On the other hand, you could save a child or children, now or in the future, some considerable distress. They are totally vulnerable, and unable to speak for themselves.

HEREDITY AND ENVIRONMENT

The nature/nurture argument is both an extension to the developmental theories already referred to and a foundation for the chapters which follow, and practice recommended therein. Why are some people simply better at some things than others? Given a similar environment to Bjorn Borg could any average young boy develop into such a tennis champion, or was something 'born in him'?

Nature

Every human being has potential which is never realised, due partly to the restrictions of opportunity. But offered equal opportunity and environment, achievements still vary considerably. Each person is a combination of that which nature has passed on, through parents, grandparents and other ancestors, together with that which the environment has caused. In considering both, the moment of influence commences at conception though before this an environmental and genetic pattern is to some extent prepared and poised for action. It is at the moment of fertilization that some decisions are made, which will be discussed later when looking at the genetic story. The developmental school of thought interprets the unfolding of personality and thought processes according to a predetermined biological pattern, earlier referred to as developmental time capsules. As mentioned, Freud's and Piaget's theories would both identify with this basic philosophy. Behaviour would be interpreted through natural inheritance, rather than the result of external influences.

Nurture

It has been claimed that any infant who presented normal, healthy characteristics, could be taken and prepared to become whatever was chosen, doctor, lawyer, artist, beggar or thief. Ignatious Loyola, a Jesuit priest, made a claim which reflects a similar philosophy, saying, 'Give me the child until he is seven, and I will show you the man'. Not only was he emphasizing the value and importance of early development and external influences, but he indicated these were irreversible to some extent.

Students of the behavioural school believe manipulation and control of the child's environment is sufficient to cause development to follow a desired pattern. The recorded incidence of children in some orphanages earlier this century support this view. They were well cared for physically, but offered no stimulation, intellectually or emotionally, they failed to thrive in any area of development. This serves as a clear illustration of environmental influence.

It has been recognised that a rare condition known as *psychosocial dwarfism*, stunted growth due to emotional starvation, is just cause for possible legal action. A case has been found proved with a 5-year-old girl taken into care along with her sister, aged 4, and a brother, aged 2.

The 5-year-old was the size of an average toddler, having the bone age of 2½ years. The siblings seemed to have developed normally. The doctor concerned with the case stated conclusively that the little girl was a victim of emotional neglect. This type of case is obviously controversial, as are any which deal with alleged ill-treatment, which cannot be easily proved by observable evidence such as a direct injury.

Another interesting example is that of the young girls reared by wolves in India, early this century, who displayed no human behavioural characteristics. Although attempts were made to socialize these girls, these were unsuccessful. Both died prematurely of suspected kidney failure, thought to be partly attributable to their intolerance of a normal human diet. The girls had been reared on raw meat.

Nature versus nurture

Basically, if one polarizes the argument of nature versus nurture, one preferring the theory that individual behaviour is the result of genetic endowment, the other, that it is the result of environmental influences, there is a sound argument for deciding a balance between the two is more acceptable. If the extremes are considered, you may appreciate the problem in accepting either, without modification. For example, if a child was gifted in a specific area such as music or art. At the extreme, a behaviourist would ascribe the skill to the presence of music in the environment, and an opportunity or persuasion to practise such skill. A developmentalist may claim the child was bound to be musical due to similarly endowed parents or grandparents. It could probably be accepted that either situation without the other would prevent such development in the child. It is fairly clear, however, that this would be most unlikely to happen, and therefore theories are difficult to prove or refute when they involve young children. Some adults claim to be 'tone deaf', but many musicians insist there is no such condition, and any ear can be trained to be sensitive to pitch. To which school of thought would these individuals belong?

If you consider yourself for a few minutes, think about your personal characteristics and skills. How many can you honestly blame, or thank, your ancestors for which cannot be helped? You may find on closer examination there are many that could be modified by external influences, or even internal motivation. If the latter is the case, from where does the drive to change come? Was it born in you, or did some influence cause it to develop? Now the two, nature and nurture, heredity and environment can be seen to be inextricably linked.

One interesting situation where biological inheritance is confirmed or confused through external influence and environment is that of sexual stereotyping. Almost unconsciously behaviour towards, and preparation of the environment for, boys and girls, differs. In the vast majority of cases the experience is supportive, and problems are few. One only has to listen to an adult, however, who has experienced a sexual identity crisis, e.g. a sex change, to appreciate the trauma of being treated as the sex with which he/she was unable to identify. This mismatch between biological inheritance and external influence often leads to serious psychological disorder.

It is presented, however, that the solution does not necessarily lie in absolute parallel treatment of both boys and girls at all times. Cultural expectations have much to do with sexual acceptance. For example it is totally acceptable for a little girl to be termed a *tomboy*, but embarrassing for a boy to be termed a *cissy*. Girls may play with cars, but it is still cause for attention if a boy carries a doll, he may however carry a teddy-bear. He may have carried a gollywog until they were 'discontinued', the manufacturers guilty of race discrimination.

PRACTICAL CHILD CARE

Take your initial interest in young children further, learn all you can about them, both by reading, and listening to what others have to say. Observe carefully, and record intelligently, both on paper, and in your memory. Place importance on the setting and maintaining of the highest standards you can possibly achieve in any given situation. Keep a sensible balance between attention to routine and hygiene, and what really matters in the interests of the children. It is not necessary to sacrifice one for the other, but to be alert to the opportunity for flexibility. The chapters which follow should act as a basic survival kit for all those embarking on a career in child care, or seriously thinking of taking such a step. It has clearly not been possible to cover in detail all the areas presented, but those which the reader finds most interesting should be followed up by further reading.

Chapter 2
Conception Through to Birth

The recipe for what becomes one of the most complex and wondrous results of nature—a human life—is relatively simple in biological terms. Two living cells fuse to become a single cell, which in turn divides into 2, then 4, and 8, and so on, until within the space of 8 weeks a perfect tiny human being is formed. This must be one of the most awesome miracles of nature. The two cells which predetermine this amazing pattern of growth come, one from the mother, and one from the father of the child. The mother's eggs, or *ova*, are present in her body when she is born, and she may have around 400,000. By the time she reaches adolescence this figure will probably have been reduced to about 10,000. Less than 500 ova are likely to reach maturity. Once a young women starts to menstruate, there will normally be one ovum released each 28 days or so. Each ovum is a potential baby. In contrast, the male, from puberty may well produce 200 million sperm each day. Each one of these may be a candidate for fertilization with the woman's ova.

Each ovum and sperm, although complete cells, contains only 23 chromosomes, which is exactly half the number contained in all other body cells. These chromosomes carry the hereditary material which at conception determines much of the future physical and mental composition of the created human life. How much is still open to argument, but such things as colour of eyes and hair and skin are determined at this moment. The cell which is thus formed has 46 chromosomes. It is interesting to note that chickens cells have 76, mice 40, and bees 16. These could be more accurately described as *pairs* of 23, 38, 20, and 8.

If nature makes a mistake and an extra chromosome appears the condition known as Down's syndrome occurs. This can now be detected by amniocentesis, a drawing off of some amniotic fluid which surrounds the fetus in which the chromosome patterning can be observed. A termination of pregnancy is usually offered if an abnormality such as Down's syndrome is diagnosed.

CONDITIONS FOR CONCEPTION

It has been mentioned that the rate of growth during the first few weeks of life is phenomenal. In order for this to happen certain conditions are desirable. These may be considered under the headings physical, emotional, social and intellectual.

Physical

Under the heading physical, both the human factor and physical environment are important. The mother and father should be fit and healthy before conception of their child. The mother especially should make an extra effort to ensure that she is able to provide the best possible environment for the unborn child. The fetus will need nourishment throughout a period of rapid and vital growth, and will take what he or she needs. If the mother is deficient in such things as vitamins or minerals, she will suffer, as well as the baby. There is certainly no need to 'eat for two' but a need to eat sensibly and healthily, maybe establishing a better pattern which could last for much longer than 9 months.

One consideration is that of weight gain, which should be carefully monitored. At each antenatal check the mother will be weighed and a certain gain is acceptable. It is quite easy to keep this gain down, without any elaborate dieting, and still remain happy and healthy. In fact the mother will often feel much better if she is lighter. She is able to move with more ease and grace, and this tends to make her feel younger and more attractive. It is the onlooker who very frequently observes that a pregnant woman looks particularly beautiful. She herself may well feel ugly and ungainly.

Smoking is harmful normally, but especially so to an unborn baby. A mother who smokes heavily runs the serious risk of damaging her child's respiratory system and his or her chances of achieving a potential birth weight. If she continues to smoke after the birth of her baby, the baby will become a secondary smoker (see Fig. 2.1),

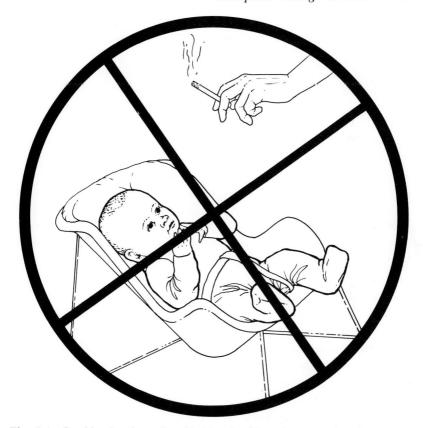

Fig. 2.1   Smoking is a hazard and babies should not be exposed to the waste it produces.

breathing the secondhand smoke around, together with a reduction of oxygen and the attendant bacteria and airborne infections.

Drinking alcohol is permissable in moderation. It is difficult to suggest how much, but it is one of those cases in which common-sense should prevail. Certain drinks such as Guinness or stout are sometimes recommended as beneficial for nursing mothers. They contain many nutrients and a considerable amount of iron. Other drinks which are very fizzy can upset the breastfed baby.

Clothing for the expectant mother can be purchased from many stores and through catalogues, and some of the designs are most attractive. It is fairly simple to make maternity clothes, and due to the relatively short life of these, cheaper materials may be chosen. Even though a woman may intend to have more than one child she will usually wish to have new maternity clothes. Trousers are very popular now with many young mothers. Shoes should obviously be comfortable, well-fitting and attractive. It is not necessary to wear flat shoes, a small heel is much more suitable. A high heel will obviously put more strain on the leg and back muscles affecting posture and is not advisable.

Rest and sleep are important too, and within the range of normal requirements, the expectant mother will know when she needs extra rest and sleep. She should respond to the messages from her body and mind. An afternoon nap is a luxury to experience before becoming a mother. Afterwards it may not be so easy. Generally an expectant mother should look and feel particularly well during the middle part of pregnancy. Morning sickness, if experienced, should have disappeared and the tedious inconveniences of the last couple of weeks or so, are still to come.

She should be encouraged to pay special attention to her appearance, clothing, hair, and make-up, if normally used. The skin may be especially clear, the hair especially manageable, this is nature's way of expressing its well being.

During the months of pregnancy most parents and their close relatives enjoy preparing the environment for the baby. The knitting needles are active and sometimes a room can be specially decorated and furnished, usually using colours and patterns suitable for either a boy or girl. It is a good idea not to choose items which reflect babyhood exclusively. Within a short time babies become toddlers, and then young school children. There are furnishings and furniture which can be adapted easily. One firm manufactures a cot, which becomes a first bed, for instance. The room should be interesting for the baby, mobiles are attractive and some produce light or have musical chimes. Pictures on the walls can be changed from time to time if posters are used, or even wrapping paper or magazine cutouts.

Heating in the room should be available, radiators as part of a central heating system or storage radiators are safe and effective. Wall heaters of the radiant type should be mounted at a safe height.

Paraffin heaters should always be avoided, as they produce a great amount of atmospheric moisture and have caused fires involving tragic loss of life. It is usually unnecessary to keep heating on during the night, unless night feeds are still required and the mother or nurse feels that she needs this comfort. Cots and prams should carry the British Standards specifications approved label, as should other items such as safety seats for cars. This ensures that the goods have been rigorously tested for safety and may be recommended. For example, some continental cots had space for a baby to slip and be trapped between the mattress and frame of the cot. If holidaying abroad in an hotel or rented accommodation, it is a point worth checking.

Emotional

The *emotional* environment for the expected child should be carefully planned. Ideally, every child should be a wanted child, arriving for two stable and loving people, secure in their own relationship with each other. This is not always the case, but many situations which do not come up to the ideal, provide very satisfactory environments for the baby. The most important factor being that of love and security, either with parent, parents or substitutes.

Child abuse often arises from a loving situation suffering from lack of support and information. There is often a fine line between hitting, and not hitting a child. One mother may have the knowledge that will prevent her from losing control. For example, a small child in a tantrum will sometimes become calm and cooperative if suitably distracted. Another successful method of calming, if at home, is to run a bath of warm water, put some toys in with the child and wait! It really can work. So the mother, for her own sake and for the child, should learn about human development, and find out where she can go for advice. Armed with this information she will be better prepared for the arrival of her child for whom she will probably be totally responsible for most of the early years, for most part of each day.

Social and intellectual

Obviously there is no direct social or intellectual link between the unborn child and the outside world. The fact that an expectant mother has a happy social life will ensure contact with a variety of people who are available to share both hopes and fears. Loneliness can give rise to anxieties which may well develop disproportionately with stress symptoms being displayed. Such symptoms as insomnia, inappropriate eating habits, smoking, drinking, agrophobia, all have a negative influence on the developing fetus.

It has been said that diet can affect the intellectual development of the unborn child. Certainly mothers suffering severe malnutrition tend to produce babies whose developmental pattern lags behind the norm, more than is acceptable. It is worth noting that such children will usually be nurtured in a deprived environment and this is responsible for the slower rate of growth in physical and intellectual areas particularly. Hidden malnutrition occurs when food is adequate, but infection is uncontrolled. This can result in conditions such as chronic diarrhoea, when nourishment is not retained within the body systems. Dehydration will cause death within hours once 10 % of the body weight has been lost.

It has been postulated that following chosen intellectual activities can predetermine a positive tendency in the unborn child. By the expectant mother listening to classical music, the fetus will be influenced, resulting in a child musically orientated, even predisposed to a particular skill. This is an interesting hypothesis, but has yet to be proved.

There is a positive link between the intelligence of natural families and the tendency for the children to reflect the abilities of their parents. It is not accepted that such a theory is inviolable, but merely that this tendency exists, and is almost certainly due to a mixture of genetic and environmental factors.

PREPARATION FOR BIRTH

The layette

The following are necessary, but most new babies are considerably over provided for, and second size clothes are needed very quickly. *Three vests*—soft fine wool, or a wool/nylon mixture—are needed.

Six 'babygros' which should *fit* without stretching, especially over the feet. Growing toes can easily be malformed with the pressure of small socks or babygros. Sizes must be checked regularly. *Plastic pants* and *six matinee jackets* or cardigans. Avoiding 'lacy' patterns in which fingers can get entangled. Ribbons may cause similar problems. *Three nightdresses*, if these are preferred to babygros for sleeping.

Dresses and romper suits are so appealing that few can resist buying them, but they are not absolutely necessary for the first few weeks. Bootees, mittens and hats are unnecessary for the new arrival, but are usually provided in profusion by friends and relatives.

Nappies are probably the most important item. They are in constant use over a relatively long period, longer than any other item of baby clothing. Depending on how often washing can be done, and on the drying facilities, the quantity required will be assessed. It is better to have a few extra, than run the risk of finding no clean dry nappies. Anything between two and four dozen terry towelling nappies may be the right amount, according to the criteria mentioned. Although it may seem a dull purchase, the mother should buy the best quality that she can afford. A good supply of liners which allow moisture to pass through, but keep a dry surface in contact with the baby's skin is very sensible. Gauze or muslin nappies are much softer and less bulky and may well be preferred whilst the baby is very small. These dry very quickly, and it is much better to dry outside if possible for all types of nappy. The fabric smells fresh and feels soft. When dried inside, the difference is quite noticeable, and drying on radiators, or in front of direct heat results in a harder, rougher texture. This of course is an aggravation to the baby's skin and may well cause soreness.

Fabric softeners are inexpensive to buy, easy to use and are effective. The rinsed clothes retain a pleasant scent and are 'springy' and soft. It should be noted that some products may cause some adverse skin conditions to erupt when the laundered articles are in contact with skins sensitive to a particular chemical.

Disposable nappies are relatively expensive, but there is a saving over laundry costs. Most mothers and fathers find them invaluable on journeys and on holiday.

FROM CONCEPTION

Whilst preparations are going on, the cause of all the activity is developing with the weeks dating from conception.

Two to three weeks. The embryo starts to form into an animal shape and measures about 2 mm (0.5 inch). A digestive tract may be identified and due to the unique chromosome pattern established, there is already an individual male or female.

Four weeks. The embryo is approximately 3 mm long or a little more. It is worth noting that this is an increase of about 50 % in a week or so. The head and spinal cord are visible, as are the buds which will become arms and legs. Blood is now flowing through tiny veins and arteries. When so much has already happened the mother will most likely not even be certain whether she is pregnant or not. One of the obvious dangers is that she may inadvertently take a drug potentially harmful to her child. The taking of thalidomide illustrates the possible interference at a very early stage of development when limbs are simply small buds. The earlier the influence the deeper and more comprehensive the damage. This works in reverse, and if the baby develops for the first 3-4 months in an ideal environment, his or her chances of being born perfectly healthy are very strong.

Five weeks. Cell specialization now occurs.

Eight weeks. The length of the embryo is approximately 3 cm (1.25 inches). This tiny being now has established eyes, ears, mouth (which opens), skull, nose, functioning liver, secreting bile, a heart with a basic beat, and a circulatory system. The arms and legs, fingers and toes are jointed although bud-like and webbed, bones and spinal cord, and a tail are present. The tail will have begun to reduce now, after reaching its maximum length at about 6 weeks. The head is approximately half the body size, becoming about a quarter at birth.

Another interesting point is that the eyes move forwards during this period from the side of the head towards their final familiar position at the front. There is still no visible difference between the sexes. From 8 weeks to birth the embryo is known as a fetus. The whole fetal period is one of elaboration and refinement of the pattern laid down in the first 8 weeks. The importance of this 2 month period cannot be overemphasized.

Twelve weeks. The fetal length is about 7.5 cm (3 inches), weighing about 20 g (.66 oz). The face is becoming more human-like, although the eyes are still fused closed. Fingernails and toenails appear, and sexual identification may be possible although any difference at this stage is slight to the observer, even though he or she may be an expert. This does not mean that there is doubt about the sex. The chromosome pattern will have determined this at conception. A female has two pairs of X chromosomes, a male has one X and one Y. At the moment of fertilization, it depends whether the X or the Y carrying sperm fuses with the femal ovum, which of course must be X. Half the sperm carry each type, X or Y. Before it was understood that the mother could not be responsible for the sex of the child, mothers were blamed for 'not giving the father a son'. Henry the Eighth is a good illustration of this ignorance.

Sixteen weeks. The weight now is about 115 g (about 4 oz). The mother may detect some movement, it is at first rather like a fluttering sensation, and can be mistaken for wind. After a few days, however, there is little doubt that this is a unique experience. There is no cause for concern if movement is not felt until a couple of weeks later. All stages of development are variable, and milestones mentioned will always reflect a norm. Added to this there may be some confusion about the date of conception. Once again a variation around the expected date of arrival of a baby must be allowed for. This gives the mother a flexible approach to her expected date of confinement, avoiding if possible the sense of depression and anticlimax if she happens to be overdue. During the fourth month, movements of the fetus may be detected by stethoscope, and if desirable observed by electronic sonar, displayed on a screen similar to a television. This method of observation is used especially if there is some concern over the rate of growth, or if there is some chance of more than one baby developing.

The fetus may swallow, purely a reflexive act, ingesting small amounts of amniotic fluid. If there appears to be too much of this fluid, saccharine has been injected into the amnion, thus stimulating the fetus into swallowing more, which may then be disposed of through the placenta (Barth 1953). This is particularly interesting as it does indicate an ability to discriminate and prefer the sweeter taste.

Research which supports that the fetus can hear was carried out in Japan. Babies of mothers who lived in noisy conditions before their birth tended to tolerate such conditions after birth. The group who were exposed to loud aircraft noise, during the first half of pregnancy, were twice as likely as the other group not so exposed, to sleep through similar loud sounds after birth. The more that is learned about human development the more important the first 3-4 months become. Some believe that listening to certain music during their pregnancy will cause their child to develop a love or even skill for such music later in life.

Twenty weeks. The weight is about 310 g (11 oz) and the length about 25 cm (10 inches). Hair begins to appear on the body of the fetus who had become distinctly humanoid in appearance. This downy covering has usually disappeared by the end of pregnancy, but some babies may be born with such hair on parts of their body. It can be rather alarming for the mother, but is just another normal stage of development taking a little longer than the familiar norm.

Pictures taken inside the womb during this period have shown the fetus with a thumb in the mouth, apparently sucking. This may or may not be accidental, but such photographs are universally appealing.

Twenty-four weeks. The weight is about 570 g (20 oz). At this stage the fetus is making breathing movements and although survival is rare, if born now, such events have been recorded. The smallest baby known to survive was born in 1937 and weighed 460 g (16 oz). At the other end of the scale, birth weights of over 9 kg (20 lb) have been recorded.

The eyelids separate during the sixth month, so the eyes will open and close. The fine hair of eyebrows and lashes may appear. By the end of the sixth month, all the essential physiological elements are established as the fetus settles down to a period of growth and strengthening. All the basic systems of respiration, circulation, digestion, elimination, and the neurological area must be poised for independent action at birth. Such systems are supported in the womb and have to make the transition quite suddenly after a few hours of the intense hard work of being born.

Twenty-eight weeks. At this point independent survival is likely, given the skilled care of a special baby unit and given that the fetus has developed normally and that the mother is fit and healthy, free from any effects of harmful drugs, an excess of alcohol, or smoking —any of these will reduce the baby's chances of survival. The movements of the fetus are quite distinct now, and there will probably be a pattern of activity and rest over the 24-hour cycle. Some mothers find that when they have managed to have an early night, the baby becomes particularly athletic. It seems that already there is a display of temperament, some mothers have such a peaceful time, they begin to wonder if the baby is alive. The doctor or midwife will soon confirm this.

Twenty-eight to forty weeks. This 12-week period often brings tedious inconveniences for the mother as her child concentrates on growing, perhaps increasing considerably in weight. Normally the total weight gain during pregnancy should not exceed 10 kg, although some mothers put on as much as 20-25 kg (44-55 lbs). This is not good for either the baby or the mother. The extra weight is difficult to lose after the birth and cannot benefit the baby in any way during the antenatal period.

The fetus is engaged in rehearsals for independent life. Babies once born need to suck in order to survive so they practise during this stage on their fingers and thumbs; they will need to breathe, so the necessary movements are made although of course no air is present. They need to eliminate so the bladder will fill and empty. The bowels will function after birth. Physically, apart from fatty layers being laid down so forming the healthy familiar new-born shape, the baby may arrive requiring a hair cut, with toenails and fingernails too long.

Antenatal check-ups

Parallel to the development of the baby, the mother will undergo regular antenatal check-ups, therefore ensuring a trouble-free period for both the baby and herself.

Once a pregnancy has been diagnosed, usually confirmed after missing a second period, or as a result of a special test if preferred, many decisions are made. These would be made between mother and doctor with the support and knowledge of the father if appropriate. Most pregnancies are confirmed with the delight of the parents. Some, however, may not be welcome for medical or social reasons, and the first decision may be whether to seek a termination. This will be discussed as a possiblity to victims of rape at one extreme, to single mothers, mothers of large families, those carrying hereditary diseases and those whose babies appear to be developing in an abnormal pattern, such as spina bifida or Down's syndrome.

Sometimes a spontaneous abortion will occur during the first 3-3½ months, due to severe abnormality. At other times there appears to be no clear cause for such an event.

Another decision is tentatively made, about whether the confinement will take place in hospital or at home. Most doctors recommend that a first, fourth and subsequent baby, a baby of a mother over 30, and understandably multiple birth shall take place in hospital. Expert skills are available should any complication arise, and all being well the mother and her child can be safely home in 48 hours. There is a strong body of opinion in favour of home confinements and the trend towards requesting such a service is growing. Many mothers quite logically feel they will be more secure and less anxious in their own home, in familiar surroundings, and with their immediate family. Where a domiciliary midwife service is available, and the 9 months of pregnancy have been straightforward and happy, the doctor may well be very supportive. For the first few months the mother will be asked to visit her doctor or clinic every 4 weeks or so. At 6 months probably fortnightly, and each week during the last month. She can of course see her doctor at any time, if she has any worries about herself or her baby. At each visit there will be a basic procedure involving simple physical tests. At the first visit a thorough check will be made, and a brief history recorded. If this is carefully documented the doctor will at this early stage be able to identify any area of possible concern. For instance a history of kidney disease could cause problems, due to the fact that these organs must work especially well during pregnancy.

ROUTINE TESTS

Weight changes should be kept under control; being underweight is as important an indication of the physical and mental condition as being overweight. If too much extra weight is acquired as well as putting strain on the body systems, it is more difficult to lose after the baby is born. It is possible to gain as little as 5.5-7 kg (12-14 lb) and have a perfectly healthy baby and mother. Some mothers increase their weight by as much as 19 kg (42 lb). It is a question of habit, and common sense, as to how much or how little an individual gains.

The presence of protein in the *urine* may indicate a rise in the load of waste products, from the mother's own body and her baby's. If she is unable to excrete these efficiently they build up causing poisoning and a condition know as eclampsia may result. Eclampsia may cause convulsions and this can damage the baby, who may be born prematurely. Cutting down on salt in the diet or avoiding it altogether as an additive, helps the elimination of toxic substances from the body.

Blood pressure will be taken at every check-up, as a rise will indicate that all is not well. A period of rest in or out of hospital often solves such a problem.

The *baby's heart* will be listened to as soon as possible and the doctor will be able to tell by palpating the abdomen that the fetus is growing as it should. Amniocentesis, testing of the amniotic fluid surrounding the fetus, is carried out if the doctor considers it to be advisable. This will normally be recommended, as mentioned earlier, for older mothers or when there is a risk of abnormality. It is the skin cells shed from the baby which are examined.

A sample of *blood* will be taken initially and then maybe once or twice during the pregnancy. A mother may need extra iron and sometimes it is prescribed as routine. Iron, however, can be a contributory cause for constipation which is often an inconvenience during pregnancy. The mother may need to compensate not by taking laxatives, but by eating more roughage and fresh fruit and by increasing her fluid intake.

At each check-up, hopefully there will be time for the mother to talk quite freely about her anxieties, however trivial they may seem.

Most worries can be allayed very easily and it is most important that she should be content and free from stress, as far as possible. Unfortunately some clinics' procedures cause the situation, where the mother sees many different doctors and is conveyed through the process of basic routine checks with the minimum of dignity and sensitivity. If general practitioners are prepared to hold their own clinics for expectant mothers they can obviously build up the sort of relationship one would look for between patient and doctor.

LABOUR

At forty weeks, normally within a few days either side of the date offered to the mother as her expected date of confinement, the baby will be born. In most cases the birth will be a natural process, perhaps with the help of some pain reducing drugs.

This normality will be looked at, before some attention is paid to events causing problems, involving more medical intervention.

First stage

The term *labour* reflects very accurately that the mother and baby have to contribute considerable energy and effort into the birth process. The mother may have any of the following indications that the first stage of labour is commencing.

A show, a blood-stained discharge consisting mainly of mucus, which plugs the cervix and is now released as the neck of this organ begins to dilate.

A backache, a dull ache low in the back which tends to travel round towards the abdomen is sometimes a fairly reliable first sign. It should be noted that these sensations can become quite defined and then fade away. Some mothers do in fact find themselves in hospital experiencing regular sensations which disappear altogether. It is quite an anticlimax and can be demoralizing and depressing especially for the mother close to her expected date.

The *rupture of membranes* is the spontaneous breaking of the membrane holding the fluid surrounding the fetus. The release of this amniotic fluid can be totally unexpected, unheralded by any other sign. In fact if the mother has been passing water at frequent intervals, and is unable to control her bladder very efficiently, she may confuse the rupture of the membrane with temporary incontinence. This sign does not leave any doubt that labour has started. Once it is established that the first stage has commenced, usually by confirming the regularity of contractions, the mother can prepare herself accordingly. She may need to make arrangements already rehearsed, for contacting husband, relatives, hospital, midwife or for children to be cared for until relatives take over. If going into hospital, transport will be required, and packed case remembered.

Certain procedures will take place if time allows, although not all midwives or hospitals follow the same pattern. The mother may be shaved, have a bath and/or an enema. The latter removes any possible obstacle to the easy passage of the baby down the birth canal. If the rectum is not empty it may be spontaneously evacuated during the second stage of labour which causes an inconvenience. Once the cervix is fully dilated the mother will probably have had the opportunity to practise her relaxation and breathing exercises learned at antenatal classes.

Second stage

The second stage of labour begins when the mother may feel a compelling urge to push or bear down. The doctor or midwife may say 'push now' or 'don't push now'. This is not an easy direction to follow as the whole body seems to be taken over by a greater force, which insists that every conceivable effort is put into the exercise of pushing. This second stage can last anything from a few minutes to an hour or two. In the latter situation the mother can become so tired that she finds it more and more difficult to participate actively and cooperatively with those caring for her. It is now that she needs the help and encouragement her partner can offer. If he can be present during the first and second stages of labour, the mother will appreciate his support and love which no-one else can offer her.

At the height of a contraction the head usually appears, and the baby may be born during the next couple of minutes. Sometimes the membrane surrounding the vagina will tear due to the demands made upon it to stretch. An episiotomy may then be performed which means making a small neat incision to allow the head to emerge. This is a painless procedure and avoids a jagged tear which will be more difficult to repair efficiently. Once the head is through, the shoulders emerge and a skilful turn results in the appearance of the complete baby. Now the mother's work is over for the time being. She can see her baby, know its sex, and feel its warm, wet and probably bloody body. All being well, she can hold the baby close to her and inspect every tiny finger and toe, wondering at this very personal miracle of nature. The expression which passes between mother and father at this moment has to be seen to be believed.

Although one appreciates the beauty of the moment, it is also very important, to the initial bonding between mother and child, that this physical contact should take place. If separation occurs for some unavoidable reason, that moment is lost, and it has been said that there is sometimes a difficulty in the establishing of this bond, and feelings of rejection have been recorded.

Final stage

The final stage of labour is the expulsion of the afterbirth, its job completed satisfactorily. It usually comes away with a couple of contractions and normally presents in one complete 'parcel'. The doctor or midwife will check that no part is missing, and the birth process is complete.

The baby will be bathed and given an initial check-over, confirming in most cases, that he or she is normal and healthy.

The mother will be washed and if necessary any repairs to her vagina will be carried out now. Mothers like to have their babies with them, especially during the first few hours. During this time they will indulge themselves in simply looking at their baby and maybe touching him or her every few minutes. This period is vitally important, it is the actual laying of foundations for future relationships, and the personal reinforcement of the event which has taken place. It represents a complete change of emotional life.

POSSIBLE COMPLICATIONS

Complications do sometimes arise, and it will be useful to look at a few of the more familiar ones.

Premature or low weight babies

A baby is termed premature if he or she weighs less than 2.5 kg (5.5 lb). The definition therefore relates to weight only, and not maturity. A full-term baby may weigh under the prescribed weight, and will be treated as premature, and given special care.

The causes for small babies may be genetic, or environmental. The latter could be due to lack of nourishment in the womb, or heavy smoking by the mother. Twins are often smaller than the average baby, simply due to the fact that there are two drawing on the same resources and they are often born early, due to their combined size triggering off an early labour. As mentioned earlier, labour may start sooner than it should due to illness or disease.

Multiple births

Apart from the sensational multiple births resulting from the administration of fertility drugs, the events of twins and triplets are not rare. Twins in fact are not a remarkable event. They may be identical, in which case they develop using the same genetic code and from a single fertilized cell. Fraternal twins develop independently and have similarities equal to those of any brothers and sisters. A set of triplets may consist of one set of identical twins and a third fraternal brother or sister. When more than one baby shares the mother's womb, it is quite common for one to present its head downwards correctly positioned for birth, and for the other to present the bottom, or be in the breech position. Although a single baby can often be persuaded to turn round by gentle manipulation, this is not as easy with twins or any multiple pregnancy.

The doctor may decide to carry out a caesarean section. This is usually, but not always, carried out under a general anaesthetic.

The surgeon makes an incision and enters the womb through the abdomen and lifts the baby out. Other situations which may indicate that caesarian section is to be considered are, when a mother has a weak heart and should not exert herself as in labour, when the pelvis is very small and the baby seems to be large enough to cause problems in passing through, when labour has been too prolonged and there is indication that the baby is becoming distressed. This will be shown on the display screen linked to the apparatus recording the condition of the baby, which is often monitored during labour or the greatest part of the process.

Forceps delivery

Forceps are used as an aid to natural birth, when labour slows down and the mother is unable to 'bear' down effectively. They are placed round the head of the baby and during the period of contraction will carefully ease the head through into the world. Marks may be visible on the head but fade quite quickly. The mother should be reassured of this as it may be upsetting for her to see these marks, which in appearance look as though they must hurt the baby, which of course they don't.

THE NEW BORN BABY

The newborn tends to look rather like any other at first and so is carefully labelled. Mothers will often be able to identify their own child within a day or two, just by looking at the face and head, but the following is a general guide to appearance and abilities.

Appearance

SHAPE

The newborn is rather an amusing shape. His or her head is about a quarter of the body length, and can often be very asymmetrical. The face is wrinkled, the nose flat, and the expression is often one of disgruntlement. The newborn has a large abdomen with skinny buttocks, legs, and arms in comparison. The neck is almost nonexistent, and often one hears the baby being resembled to grandparents or referred to as a 'little old man'.

BONES

The bones of the skull have to complete their growth, having left a central gap on the top of the head to allow for some pressure during birth. The gap at the front is diamond shaped and called the *anterior fontanelle*, through it a pulsating can often be observed. The gap at the back, the *posterior fontanelle*, is so small it cannot always be detected. These gaps do not represent weakness and the mother should not avoid proper washing of this area. Avoidance or neglect can result in cradle cap, a thick yellowy crust of solid scurf. This can be treated very effectively but does look unsightly and can upset the mother.

GENITALS

The genitals may be enlarged due to hormones passing through the placenta to the baby. Baby boys or girls may have tiny 'breasts' and girls may have slight discharge from the vagina. All such effects will usually disappear within the first week.

SKIN

Dry, blotchy or peeling skin may be observed. There may be little white spots on and around the nose or tiny red ones around the neck. The only cause for concern is an infected spot, the others will disappear, and if the 'nappy' area becomes sore. The small spots inside the mouth of a grey yellowy colour are called 'Epstein's pearls' and these too disappear in a few weeks.

At first every sound made by the baby is noticed by the mother. She will be amused by sneezes, hiccoughs, and yawns, concerned about snuffles and changes in breathing. She may even check during the longest period of sleep that the baby is in fact still alive and breathing, his or her respiration is more shallow and the rate is rapid, sometimes alarmingly so, to the new mother. Skin colour is the first sign of jaundice. The newborn often develops what is termed 'normal' or physiological jaundice, which disappears without treatment within a few days. The doctor will keep the baby under close observation as a severe case can cause brain damage.

Abilities

The new baby has a very wide range of abilities, even though he or she is totally dependent on those who care for him or her, and would die without such care.

REFLEXES

The newborn possess senses which operate more efficiently than was realized until recently. It is obvious that the baby can hear, as the startle reflex can be observed when a sudden sound is produced. A similar action is seen when a baby is threatened with being dropped, throwing his or her arms out in a wide movement and bringing them back. Another reflex, that of swallowing, has been mentioned with reference to fetal development. That of 'rooting' is displayed when the baby searches for food by nuzzling his or her mother, and sometimes with others who handle him or her. The head will also turn in the direction of a touch on the check. All normal babies suck immediately after birth if put to the breast, some efficiently, others in a rather experimental way. This is not learned behaviour but another reflexive action.

Another interesting reflex is that of walking movements, if the baby is held in an upright position, over a firm surface. Grasping is also a strong action, strong enough to support the whole weight of the baby. If placed in water soon after birth a baby will make swimming movements, and babies have actually been born under water. One by one these reflexive behaviours die out as the more mature parts of the brain develop.

CRYING

Crying is one of the essential abilities, as this is the communication channel through which the mother can identify the expressed needs of her baby. She will become accustomed to his or her different cries and will interpret these is order to respond appropriately.

The differences may reflect pain, hunger, cold, overheating, boredom or loneliness. A baby cries for a reason, he or she is saying something, and it is the first method of communication, the first attempt to socialize. If these cries go unanswered the baby may learn to distrust his or her world, and may feel insecure and unhappy. The baby will not learn to be 'good' through being ignored, although this may appear to happen. He or she simply gives up trying and withdraws from the unsympathetic environment. The cry of a baby is not a useless activity, nor is it a way of 'exercising the lungs'.

Possible depression

At this time the mother has every reason to rejoice and be happy. It is therefore confusing and unreasonable to her if a sense of deep depression overwhelms her, and she may even have a feeling of indifference towards her baby, tending in some mothers towards temporary rejection. This beautiful defenceless human being, whose arrival she has looked forward to for so long, suddenly appears alien to her.

The best possible support is to be found either in her own mother or in a mother who has experienced such emotions and succeeded in coping with them. Only extreme cases require medical treatment. Having said this, the mother should be treated with sympathy, as these unwelcome emotions can be quite frightening.

Feeding pattern

One way of coming to terms with the new role of motherhood is to establish a successful pattern of feeding. This is always an achievement recognized by all around her, and creates a bond between mother and baby which is very difficult to define in words. The fixed eyes of the baby on the mother's eyes cause any observer to feel very much an outsider.

BREASTFEEDING

Benefits of breastfeeding are as follows. It is the final natural stage of the reproductive cycle. The sucking of the baby stimulates the uterus and it is encouraged to return to its normal size. Mothers who breastfeed tend to lose the added weight gained during pregnancy more easily and in a shorter time. Milk will be produced anyway, and must be artificially suppressed if the mother is determined not to breastfeed. The milk is presented on demand at the correct temperature, free from bacteria, of the correct constitution for a human baby, and as a bonus, carrying some valuable immunities from the mother.

The main differences in the formula of human milk as compared with cow's milk, the common substitute, are: human milk has less protein, containing less casein, the least digestible component. In a bottlefed baby these undigested curds may be observed in the stools. Human milk has a lower sodium and phosphate content, minerals which can overload the new baby's kidneys. It is fair to point out that milk formulae recommended for feeding infants are modified, and do provide an excellent recipe of nutrients if breastfeeding is not possible.

Breastfed babies do not tend to put on surplus weight, and although they may seem to vary their requirements at different times during the day, they only take what they need, no extra. The mother often seems to see an empty bottle as totally satisfactory, and is concerned if a bottle is left unfinished. Living things do not necessarily require exactly the same quantity of food each time they eat. Most importantly, breastfeeding establishes an emotional bond between mother and baby, which has a unique quality, denied to the bottlefed baby and mother. It is nourishment for body and soul. Having said this, if a mother cannot breastfeed her baby she should be encouraged to create a situation as close to the natural one as she can. Holding the baby close to her throughout feeding, not leaving its bottle propped beside the baby which is dangerous due to the possi-

bility of the baby choking, and at first, not handing the job of feeding
to others too frequently. Obviously one of the advantages of using a
bottle is that the father can be involved, and may even offer to take
care of night feeds, allowing the mother to sleep through.

Starting to breastfeed if the nipples are normal, not introverted,
ought to be fairly straightforward. Even if the mother is a little ten-
tative, the baby will usually know exactly what to do. There may not
be much milk for the first day or two, but the baby will suck the col-
ostrum secreted in small quantities. This fluid has a high protein
content, and contains some antibodies, so nourishes and protects the
baby immediately.

Pure human milk is surprisingly watery looking, and many
mothers have given up feeding their babies, because they say their
milk was 'no good'. This is simply never true, just as it is never true
that the size of a breast has anything to do with ability to breastfeed
satisfactorily. Women with very small breasts have fed their children
happily for the best part of their first year of life, alongside a satisfactory mixed diet. Incidentally, although the chances are reduced, a
mother can become pregnant whilst she is still breastfeeding. This is
one cause of a reduction in the supply of milk and a recommendation
for weaning, in order to ensure proper nourishment for the new
embryo.

Feeding on demand is often popular with breastfeeding mothers.
This need not lead to a totally haphazard lifestyle. There is always a
need for some routine, albeit a flexible one, if the rest of the family is
to live happily through the experience of having a new baby. Allow
the baby to establish his or her pattern, it will probably be 6 or 7
feeds a 24-hour cycle to begin with, the gaps being of various lengths.
Very quickly the baby will sleep much longer for the night period,
especially if fed a little later than the traditional 10.00 p.m. feed,
then the mother can look forward to her rest.

One of the biggest problems is often the tiredness of the mother.
She may be looking after other children, running the home, and getting up in the night too. If she can take short rests during the day or
have an early night, and risk being disturbed, it can make a lot of
difference. An attitude of mind can be as relaxing as actual sleep,
and if the mother accepts the temporary lack of adequate sleep philo-

sophically, the risk of it becoming a problem is greatly reduced. Although it seems to loom as a permanent way of life, nappies and sleepless nights really do become a part of personal history and survival, very quickly.

BOTTLEFEEDING

One of the benefits of bottlefeeding is that it can be shared. The mother is not tied to feeding times and the baby can be left with friends and relatives if desired. Mothers sometimes prefer to bottle-feed because they feel the need to actually see how much formula the baby has consumed.

The equipment required in order to be ready to bottle feed, should be acquired before the birth of the baby. Even mothers who intend and hope to breastfeed should have a couple of bottles in which to offer water, fruit juice, or supplementary feeds if necessary.

Equipment

1 Six bottles and caps. There is now a variety of shapes and types of bottle to choose from, and a decision will rest with the mother, according to comfort of holding, ease of cleaning, and appearance.
2 Approximately six teats or nipples. These may already be marked according to size of hole. Too big and the baby may choke; too small and the baby will become frustrated and tired, and may take in too much air. Holes may be enlarged with a hot needle, or a cross may be made with a razor.
3 Small spoon. Long handled spoon for mixing if necessary, although the method of mixing now is often by a simple shaking method.
4 Measuring scoop for milk powder. Always make sure the correct scoop is used for a particular type of formula. Always measure with care and precision. The instruction for five measures, means five level measures, not about five, not one for luck, and not one less because the tin of powder is running low. Always ensure there is a spare packet of food for the baby, and check especially before the weekend or any Bank holiday. There is no food substitute which will

satisfy the baby, and borrowing some from a neighbour may result in a strange formula causing an upset.

If a spare packet is kept watch the expiry date, and even better when used, replace it as soon as possible.

5 Measuring jug.
6 Sterilizing unit and tablets of Milton.
7 Bottle brush.

The other items will be in the kitchen normally: kettle, tray, cutlery, washing facilities for hands and utensils. A bottle warmer is useful but not essential. A jug of hot water is equally effective, but make sure the milk is tested for warmth, better to err on it being a little cool, than a little hot. In fact many babies don't seem to mind very much if the milk is a little cooler than recommended. When a few drops are shaken onto the inside of the wrist, the sensation should be one of warmth. Follow the directions of the packet of formula very carefully when making up the feed. Too concentrated a feed may cause constipation or dehydration. In some of the third world countries, the mothers are unable to read or make up the feeds correctly and have actually starved their babies.

A comfortable position for mother and baby should be found in a quiet warm place, where the process can be completed undisturbed. The presence of other people makes little difference, neither do normal household sounds, it is sudden intrusion which may cause distraction. The bottle should always be held at an angle which keeps the milk covering the feeding end completely, all the time.

Quantity

It is quite simple to work out how much milk to make up each time. A reliable guide is that recommended by many experts of 65 ml per 450 g of body weight (2½ fl oz per lb of body weight) per 24-hour cycle. About 50 calories per pound of body weight per day. As mentioned before it is unlikely that the baby will divide his or her need for nourishment equally throughout the day. For example, taking a 3.6 kg (8 lb) baby. This baby will require 500 ml (20 fl oz) during 24 hours. At this weight, he or she may be happy with five feeds of 100 ml (4 fl oz) or so. To allow for the slight fluctuations of requirements from feed to feed it may be a good idea to offer a little extra each time. The easiest way would be to make sufficient for the 24-hour period adding 16 ml (0.66 fl oz). This amount divided equally will prove a little surplus to the basic 100 ml (4 fl oz) each time, and any not used should be thrown away. It will be obvious after a short time which feeds should be larger or smaller.

The mistake of interpreting all crying as hunger must be avoided. It is very common to offer food as the universal comforter and reflect the habit that exists throughout many peoples lives, resorting to food or drink at times of stress.

General advice

Evaporated milk is suitable for small babies and again the advice must be to follow the instructions carefully.

Before preparing feeds, hands must always be washed. Keep all utensils clean and covered away from animals or other children. Bottles and teats are easily sterilized in solution using a liquid or tablet form of sterilizing agent. Again, read all the instructions carefully.

If a number of feeds are prepared at one time keep covered in the refrigerator until required.

Never leave a baby alone with a bottle propped on the pillow beside him or her. Apart from denying the emotional satisfaction the baby is entitled to, he or she can very easily choke.

If small amounts of milk are returned when the baby is rested during a feed or afterwards there is no cause for alarm. Real vomiting results in large quantities being rejected by the stomach and indicates something is wrong. A baby can very quickly become dehydrated, and vomiting should always be treated seriously. Bottlefed babies do tend to suffer from gastrointestinal disorders more than breastfed babies, another argument in support of breast-feeding.

Finally, whichever method of feeding is chosen some mothers are anxious and need support and encouragement, others have very few problems and plenty of support. Babies are tough, resilient and very demanding and most thrive successfully and happily through the inexperienced but loving care of their mothers. Most first born children bear testament to this.

Some thoughts from the *Standard,* Wednesday September 9th 1981.

'At the beginning I was terrified of him, I didn't know what to do with him, I didn't know how to hold him, how to change him or anything.

The biggest shock was the amount of time it required to look after a newborn baby. I just never dreamed that I'd be spending every waking minute and every sleeping minute just looking after him, doing one thing after another for him.'

'The first day I got home was especially bad. I found I spent most of the day weeping. I think at first there was that really over-whelming sense of responsibility, caused by the fact that they're so completely helpless. I like her but I don't like looking after her. I don't like the fact that she has to depend on me for everything. I mean you don't exist when you have a baby, do you?'

INFLUENCE ON PARENTS

The influence on the relationship between parents, of the arrival of a third member of the family and one who is so dependent, requires some understanding. The father, unless he is unusually mature and well-prepared can easily feel neglected and may display his feelings, causing the mother to feel unduly depressed and worried, when she is emotionally very vulnerable. If the father has prepared for the event properly, he will anticipate that the mother will feel anxious, at times inadequate, at times overemotional and that she will be very busy in her new role. It is a time when some young men find that they have to do the final bit of growing up themselves.

Chapter 3
Development in the First Two Years

STAGES OF DEVELOPMENT

During the first two years of life, although a baby increases considerably in size, the rate of development which took place during pregnancy is never equalled. Babies, however, are likely to double their birth weight by 6 months and treble it at a year old. During this short time they will develop the skills of mobility, communication, loving and being loved, socializing and functioning intellectually. All these are obviously interdependent and the quality of the environment, personally and structurally, will affect the rate and nature of these areas of growth.

At three months

Babies are responding to their surroundings at three months, kicking and waving their arms and bringing their hands together. Using their arms they can support their head and chest when placed on their stomach. If they are pulled up into a sitting position, their head will fall back a little. They will be able to follow movements and are particularly interested in faces, real or drawn. Mobiles are attractive to them. They will grasp an object of suitable size, and fondle the bottle or breast when feeding. They recognize the bottle and display pleasure on seeing it. They also recognize their mother's voice, and should be talked to whenever possible as they now begin to vocalize experimentally. The pattern of their first sound, or lack of it, can be the first indication of hearing loss. There are still many children who suffer from late diagnosis of such defects, and experience extensive learning difficulties in their first days at school. The periods of wakefulness extend, and there will be times when babies are particularly eager to be played with, as they learn to socialize. If they can be persuaded to be lively early in the evening, their father may have the opportunity to get to know them better. They may then be just a little more prepared for a long sleep. Obviously they should not be involved in an exciting type of play, but the value of a relationship with both parents is so important. Many fathers do not see their small babies awake at all during the week.

At six months

Growth is still taking place at quite a rate and babies may, on average, have doubled their birth weight at the end of 6 months. They will be physically individual now, and it will be easy for friends and relatives to discriminate between this particular baby and other babies. Photographs taken now will be identifiable later on.

POSTURE AND MOVEMENT

If they are pulled up into a sitting position, the head will arrive first. They will anticipate the action too by holding their hands out, and they will cooperate in dressing, although the movements will be subtle. Babies may sit for a few moments before toppling sideways. They will enjoy sitting supported in the pram, the safety harness prevents them from losing this comfortable position. They should never be left in a pram, once they have reached the stage of possibly being able to fall out. Both straps should be attached to the anchor points and then sharply tugged to test their firmness. Babies have been known to suspend themselves over one side of the pram when a strap has been carelessly fixed, or is too old to be safe. They can strangle themselves in such a way. Do not release the straps if the baby drops off to sleep, he or she may look uncomfortable, but may wake up unexpectedly and be in serious danger.

The 6-month-old will take a toy or other small object, passing it from hand to hand, maybe indicating as this early stage a preference for left or right. Babies can release their hold, and enjoy dropping things, showing no interest once the objects are out of sight. The concept of permanence is not yet established.

SPEECH

The sounds made now should be tuneful, and are often repetitive consonants such as 'da-da' and 'mum-mum'. It is interesting to look at the words used for mother and father in other countries, they usually reflect the first sounds made in infancy.

MOBILITY

The first independent action in this direction will be one of rolling over, from the stomach on to the back. At first they will not be able to reverse this movement.

TEETHING

Another outward sign of growth is that of erupted teeth or those pre-paring to show. This varies very much, and babies have been born with teeth. Normally at 6 months the two lower incisors are visible centrally placed in the gum. The two either side usually follow. Some babies unfortunately have a miserable time, others show little sign of distress or discomfort. There are gels available to rub on the gums, which seem to comfort some babies. They tend to dribble at these times and may have flushed cheeks. Once again, another natural stage of growth and development which should not give rise for undue concern. One of the dangers is that of ascribing symptoms to 'teething', e.g. loose stools, high temperatures, which may repre-sent other problems.

COLOUR OF HAIR AND EYES

Usually there will be sufficient hair on the head to indicate the colour it is going to be finally. Similarly the eyes will probably have changed from their initial baby blue.

FEEDING

Although babies will still enjoy the feed from breast or bottle, they could be happily on an established mixed diet, drinking from a cup, with just a breast or bottle feed at night.

The introduction of different textures could take place during the first month, but should be happening by the third or fourth month. Waiting longer than 6 months is inadvisable. Firstly, babies are not as adaptable to new textures the older they get, and in extreme cases of very late weaning from breast or bottle, mothers have found it very difficult indeed to make the change. Secondly, the store of iron in the baby's liver begins to run down, and no type of milk contains sufficient for the needs of growth at this stage, which is still rapid. This is why egg yolk, rich in iron, is often recommended as a suitable introduction to weaning. Other foods with high iron content are green vegetables, especially spinach, treacle or molasses, and cocoa. Liver is rich in iron, as are other meats to a lesser degree. The flavour of some types of meat, however, can be rather strong for a very young baby. Mashed chicken liver may be acceptable, as it breaks down easily. The decision when to start mixed feeding rests upon various criteria. Is the baby hungry after his or her recommended amount of milk feed? If the mother is breastfeeding has she prepared herself emotionally for the change in her baby's dependency? The contra-indications for early weaning are the expectancy of longer sleeping periods, and boredom and impatience by the mother. Mixed feeding does not guarantee the former, and the latter takes little account of the baby's needs.

The first 'solid' foods should be smooth in consistency. Cereals which are mixed with milk, or other powdered preparations, must be carefully mixed gradually introducing the fluid to the powder, not the other way round. Lumps cause problems to the baby experimenting with a new medium, and the coughing which may result is unpleasant and even frightening for the child. The golden rule of weaning is of gradually progressing from a milk diet to a mixed one. Introduce cereal or other chosen food at one mealtime for a few days. Then increase to two and then three. This will probably take a few weeks before the traditional and familiar pattern of three meals a day emerges. In addition the bedtime milk feed and early morning juice should be continued. These habits often persist happily throughout life. All hospitals offer a milky drink to patients before settling them for the night.

So from the starting point of a teaspoonful or two of smooth puree, e.g. cereal, broth, once a day. Weaning is complete when a mixed diet has been established, together with any fluid being taken from a cup.

Utensils

There are various types of spoons and 'pushers' on the market and it may be simply a question of personal preference on the part of the mother or baby which is used. For the introductory feeds a plastic spoon is often accepted more easily than a metal one, being less harsh to the teeth, especially if cold. As with fluids, although adults tend to imagine that warm food must be preferable to cold food, babies do not seem to mind. If out on a picnic or planning for a journey, it may be worth experimenting to find out if the baby will accept cold foods. If he or she will, then unopened and therefore sterile jars or tins of a proprietary baby food can be taken, making the feeding so much simpler and safer.

Food kept warm in a flask should be avoided if possible, it should be kept hot and then cooled. The favourite breeding ground for bacteria is warm, moist and oxygenated. All these conditions will prevail in a flask of warm food. Don't imagine that the name 'vacuum' flask means that the contents are in a vacuum.

With crockery, there are many attractive designs available. One good idea is that of a suction pad underneath a bowl or plate keeping it firmly in position. Be prepared for some mess, and at times whole meals being upset. It is surprising to the uninitiated how quickly a reluctant eater can remove the offending plate of food. Babies learn through experimentation, and one of the first materials to be explored is food. Allowing them to learn to be independent and keeping control of the food often creates problems. Offering some dry food, such as cubes of fried bread, small pieces of fruit or broken rusk, at the same time as the baby is being fed can be tried. They will, if in the appropriate mood, concentrate on these, and eat from the spoon held by the adult. If the babies have their own spoon they can practise with it, using just a small amount of food. The frustration of failure will not develop, as their hunger is being satisfied by the adult.

Satisfying hunger is one of the most common social activities known to man. All cultures tend to display friendship or acceptance of others, by eating and drinking with them. This is seen throughout the social hierarchy as well as across the cultures. It is difficult to accept, but easier to appreciate why such emphasis is placed on the feeding of babies and children. It is sad and unnecessary for such an activity to become of such concern to the adult that mealtimes become a battleground. Unfortunately question and answer columns in magazines tend to reflect that this happens all too frequently. The situation will be discussed in more detail (see p. 53).

What a baby eats is important, and much depends on the pattern adopted by the family. On the whole try to avoid the foods which tend to carbohydrate and sweetness. One of the main nutritional problems in the western world is that of overweight, and overweight mothers often rear similar children. For all sorts of reasons, medical, social and emotional this is most undesirable. Years ago it was the plump bonny baby who won the baby competitions, larger gains in weight were regarded as healthy development. Slim children often elicited remarks such as 'Oh, he looks as though he needs feeding up'. It would be much kinder to the children to ensure good eating habits very early in life and educate the future mothers more comprehensively on nutrition for themselves and their children.

There are still too many young children going to school in the morning without adequate nourishment to start the day, or with packets of 'junk' food to compensate. There are too many tuck shops selling useless snacks, in order to augment the school funds, and too many babies observed in their prams consuming items which have only been offered as temporary pacifiers. It is so easy to do, and once again becomes a habit expected by the child. It has been said that an overfed child lays down more fat cells than necessary, thus causing a tendency to be overweight throughout life.

At nine months

Normally babies will sit happily and in a straight backed position for some time before tiring. This point should be watched for, as they will probably be unable to voluntarily lie down. Similarly if they pull themselves up to a standing position they cannot always revert to a sitting one, and may cry quite bitterly whilst hanging on to their support, frightened to let go. Some babies are mobile now, many by crawling forwards or backwards, some by shuffling, and it has been known for babies to walk as early as this. These are usually lighter individuals, with well developed muscular systems, and a highly developed urge to explore the environment.

Another group which seem to display a rapid rate of motor development is that of black infants. Researchers have recorded an acceleration of motor development in infants studied in Uganda (Ainsworth *et al.* 1966). If the rate of such progress is determined genetically, then maybe black races simply carry a different programme. There could be an environmental reason, as the families who had become westernized, keeping their babies in cots and prams, reflect the western norm of motor development. Whether a child walks at 9 months or 19 months is of little importance, if all is normal. There may be a very good social reason for the late walker. If there is an older brother or sister prepared to bring the things the baby needs, motivation will be much less than if he or she has to reach for them.

The mother will be recognized together with other familiar members of the family, who will be greeted vocally. The infant will respond to familiar 'naming' words, i.e. 'mummy' and 'daddy', car, pram, drink. This order of understanding is reflected in first clear words which are usually of a similar category, together with such social responses as 'bye-bye'. Socially, games may now be played with the baby being an active participant. Among the most popular are hide and seek, both using objects and faces, thus illustrating the developing concept of permanence, knowing that if something vanishes from sight it still exists. Communication games using body movements are also popular, often introducing 'fun fear', e.g. 'Ride a cock horse' on the knee, simulating a fall at the appropriate moment, or 'Round and round the garden like a teddy bear'.

This attraction of self induced fear lasts into maturity, hence the popularity of horror films and some amusement park spectaculars.

One fear babies are unprepared to tolerate, is that of strangers, and if this is the case, they will be truly inconsolable until returned to a familiar person. Relatives unable to visit frequently may be rejected, and should feel no personal failure, but appreciate that the baby's obvious unhappiness is just another natural stage in his or her development.

One way the 9-month-old will communicate with strangers is by displaying the skill of letting go. Most of us are familiar with the dropped toy, which when returned to the baby will be dropped for the next sympathetic passerby. This is not only a display of muscular refinement, but of voluntary socializing.

At one year

The first birthday is in itself a milestone and a cause for celebration. In a short year from a totally dependent rather plain little scrap of humanity the baby has emerged as an attractive personable independent individual.

One-year-olds will normally be mobile by one chosen method or another. They will make reasonable attempts to feed themselves and will be able to communicate their needs and feelings in a satisfactory way. They will know their family and may feel confident with strangers in the prescence of those who are familiar to them.

SAFETY

At one year, they will follow simple directions particularly when accompanied by appropriate body language. They will be very curious and eager to explore, which as they are probably mobile gives rise to problems of safety. It is surprising how soon a baby learns to climb, and putting things out of reach does not guarantee that they will remain so. Once children are mobile they should never be left unsupervised unless they are safely in bed or strapped in their pram. Even in the pram, it is advisable to position it if possible, in such a way that it can be observed from the house. Leaving a baby unattended outside a shop should be avoided, unless the family dog is left on guard. The efficiency of the brakes on prams and push chairs should be checked at regular intervals.

A toddler should never sit on the end of a pram without someone holding the handle. They are not designed with this distribution of weight accounted for, unless they are twin prams. Another danger is that of pram seats for toddlers. Some may become dislodged when the pram is taken up or down a steep curb. If this happens it is difficult to know which to take hold of, with one hand on the handle, and toddler and seat detaching themselves. It is better to check that the type chosen can be fitted very securely.

Inside the house, plugs used to be the greatest hazard, but if the type with safety shuttering are fixed, this avoids the possibiltiy of babies pushing fingers and other items into the holes.

Most accidents to young children unfortunately take place in the home and most can be prevented. Safety in the home will be looked at more closely in Chapter 8.

FAMILY ROUTINE

One-year-olds should have adapted to the family routine. Apart from their need for more rest and sleep, it is usually unnecessary to make any special arrangements for them. They will, if meals are planned accordingly, need no special food, and will be able to join fully in family mealtimes. On the occasions when the dish is not suitable, being too highly spiced, or too oily, i.e. fatty, a few jars or tins, or a few small suitable portions kept in the freezer will keep them happy.

When Christmas arrives do not presume that the baby, or very young child will feel deprived without all the accompanying festive delights. Better to keep to the sort of food with which they are familiar. It is not a time for experimentation, or for risking a gastric upset. For everyones sake also, the familiar routine should be followed with a certain degree of flexibility or a family will become a slave to it, but within reasonable limits.

Babies and young children seem to have a sixth sense with which to diagnose the unusual, and any deviation will activate this sense. For instance, the parents are going out, and want the baby to go to sleep before they go. Even though they carefully follow the same routine as usual, there seems to be some indication, probably through communication of attitude or behaviour, which causes the baby to react and become anxious. The baby probably remains awake longer than he or she has ever done before.

LEARNING THROUGH THE SENSES

Through the senses all learning takes place. Early in life the human baby will develop more fully the senses he or she needs, and allow to become less efficient those not required. For instance blind children often develop a much more acute sense of hearing, and a finer sense of touch than sighted people.

During the first year, the senses are likely to be used in the following way.

Sight

At birth, sight is now thought to be reasonably efficient, the eyes moving together after a few days. The pupils' reaction to light also becomes efficient during the first week or so. Babies of 2 weeks old seem to be able to discriminate between colours although they could be reacting to intensity rather than actual colours (Chase 1937). Focussing on moving objects takes a little longer to develop, the optimum range for infants is about 3-4 cm (8-10 inches) which is about the distance from the mothers face of a naturally held baby whilst feeding. During the year, the baby will focus well, follow a moving object, coordinate efficiently hand and eye movement, and discriminate between people.

Smell

Little is known about the efficiency of smell, apart from the fact that strong smells will elicit some reaction. An obvious discrimination between taste could reflect some ability to smell as taste is considerably dulled if the sense of smell is malfunctioning. Another indication is that a breastfed baby knows if his or her mother is holding him or her. If the baby is nearing a feed time he or she is restless and 'roots' for nourishment. This behaviour is rarely so displayed if others are holding the baby.

Taste

There is obviously an ability to discriminate between sweetness and blandness as mentioned, during prenatal development. There is also a clear reaction to salt, as indicated by the infant during baptism, when a pinch of salt is placed on the lips or tongue. The baby doesn't seem to mind this taste, but clearly responds. During the first year preferences for tastes and textures will emerge, and should be respected. It is during this time that habits will be formed as mentioned earlier. A sweet tooth is the responsibility of the parent.

Hearing

The hearing is well-developed at birth. Proof that this is so is indicated by an increase in the rate of heartbeat monitored when a baby is exposed to sounds such as bells, rattles and squeaks. Loud sounds elicit the startle reflex, but some may not be a reliable indication of auditory functioning, as the response observed could be due to vibration.

By 6 months babies will be able to locate sound and turn their head in the right direction. By the time the first year has been completed the 1-year-olds will reflect this skill of hearing and listening through their own level of language acquisition. They should produce a pattern of various pitches and pauses, a bit like speech which could be an imaginary language, containing some familiar words. 'Babies minds are far sharper than we give them credit for. Long before they can walk or talk their brains make sense of what they see, and hear.' (Butterworth 1982). As early as 4 months they recognize their parents' voices and look towards them, even if the voice is played from a tape recorder some distance away. They also perceive objects from as early as 2 months and in some cases will find them even if they are hidden in one place after another.

The traditional idea that babies' early experiences were chaotic needed to be revised. It used to be thought that because their perception of other objects was poor babies saw themselves as the centre of the universe until they were 18 months old. It is now maintained that they realize much earlier that they are only one object in a world of objects (Butterworth 1982).

This is a clear illustration of research presenting new ideas challenging existing theories, and thus pointing out to those who study the development of children, that the answers may not all be found yet, and there is a need to approach such study with an open, flexible and enquiring mind.

Touch

As soon as the infant enters the world he or she is sensitive to touch. So important does this sense appear that premature babies have actually shown more ability and desire to thrive when placed on sheepskin than on the normal cotton sheet. As soon as the small hands reach out they begin to convey to the baby information regarding such things as texture and temperature.

By the end of the first year babies will show preference for some textures and may have adopted an article without which they will be unable to settle to sleep. This may be a toy but is often a piece of fabric. No substitute will be accepted and if it is washed it is usually rejected. Is this another indication of olfactory discrimination? It will look and feel the same, so it may be the familiar smell that is missing. The urge to touch seems to remain into maturity. People in stores, touch and feel articles for the pleasure of doing so, few women will pass through a fabric department without touching at all. Some materials seem to have a comforting property. Velvet and fur fall into this category, and cushions covered in this type of fabric are universally popular.

In contrast there are some textures which individuals can hardly bear to experience. Amongst these could be slimy surfaces, sandpaper or brushed nylon. All these have been noted as causing a negative reaction on touching. This sense does become well-developed in most adults, but those displaying an extremely highly developed sense of touch are of course readers of Braille. To one who has never felt a page of Braille it seems totally impossible that sense can be made out of what is felt beneath the fingertips. As with all categories of learning the earlier it is mastered the easier it will be, and adults going blind later in life will encounter much more difficulty in learning Braille than a young child.

The eyes can become lazy. This is why sometimes one eye will be covered if the other one has been depending too much on it. The lazy one is made to work, otherwise it will actually become less efficient on a permanent basis. Muscles which are not used also behave in this way. Getting up again after a few days in bed clearly illustrates how quickly the system is willing to prepare for retirement. At the other end of the life span it is relevant to mention that old people definitely remain physically and mentally more alert if some effort is made or there is a necessity to do so. Old people who play bingo regularly scored higher in tests for mental alertness than those who did nothing demanding similar concentration.

It should be noted that the mouth is used to experience and explore objects as much as the hands for the first few months. Gradually this will die out, although it can be observed as common behaviour in mentally retarded or disturbed adolescents and adults.

INDIVIDUALITY

Having looked fairly briefly at the first year of development it is interesting to note there are differences not only in motor development but in temperament, patterns of activity and attitudes to the world, human and structural. For instance, some babies love to be handled and cuddled, others wriggle or remain apart in the physical sense. It has been said that these differences persist throughout life and many mothers would support such a statement. The environment during the period of development covered in this chapter is second only to the prenatal situation. Much, if not all , that happens in the experience of the baby during this first year will have some effect on his or her future development: physically, socially, emotionally and intellectually.

Baby to toddler

It becomes less relevant to link ages to stages during the baby to toddler phase, the older the human being the more flexible the stages. For instance, a child may learn to read at any age from 2 ½ years, at one extreme, to 8 or 9 years at the other, and still be within an acceptable normal distribution curve. Most children will learn at about 5 or 6 years, that is, the middle of the curve.

Most individuals are sufficiently mature in the emotional sense to marry in their late teens or early twenties. Some marry successfully at 16, others wait until middle age. The older the person the less age really matters. So already development will be looked at not in stages of 3 months but in easily identifiable periods.

THE TODDLER/THE SECOND YEAR

The child will be toddling around during the second year of life, either around his or her first birthday or even approaching the second. This second year of development will be looked at as a whole with emphasis on one or two aspects. One of the main differences linked to mobility is that the environment may be explored, no longer does the environment have to come to the baby.

Their environment

The physical development of toddlers will directly relate to their ability to embark on a programme of exploration. The quality of their immediate world will influence the experiences they are offered, and determine their range of learning. The responsibility of the adult is to ensure that life is filled with a variety of 'happenings', together with interesting and stimulating materials at appropriate times. It must be appreciated that children so young still need adequate periods of rest and sleep, together with quiet times for loving and being happy, because human beings must learn these skills just as any other. It is not easy to love without ever having experienced being on the receiving end of this emotion, and mature relationships need a foundation on which to build. This foundation must be laid in very early childhood.

'Happenings' should be planned in order to expand the children's world. They will be interested in all that is going on around them and will enjoy going out for walks, during which the opportunity to talk should always be taken. It seems a pity that many prams or push chairs are constructed in such a way that the child cannot communicate directly with the adult. Opportunities to extend the social world should be created by introducing the child to others, who need not necessarily be his or her own age. Older children provide real life drama by simply playing within sight and sound. For the toddler sitting in the pram close to a playground can be entertaining and often can lead to social contacts for the mother. Being a young mother can be a very lonely life, and it is surprising and sad how many problems arise out of this loneliness.

Communication

At around 18 months of age, given adequate language experience children will begin to express themselves more skilfully, by joining words together sensibly. They will, however, seem most economic in their choice of words at the same time being clever enough to select the 'key' ones needed to convey the message. For instance, the response to 'Come on put your coat on, we're going out now' could well be 'Coat out now'. These could also be used in question form once the concept of 'coat' and 'going out' are linked. It is interesting to note how frequently the 'useful' words are selected. It would be as easy for the child to pronounce and reproduce any of the sentence, but 'on going out' is never chosen. This indicates the possibility of a genetically inherited ability to understand that language has order and must stick to certain rules.

Avoid using 'baby talk'. It is no easier to pronounce. It means that many words have to be relearned, and this seems to serve no useful purpose. Added to this there is no need to adopt a special voice, speak more loudly, or speak for a child. The latter becomes a very irritating habit, which can remain well into adolescence, causing much embarrassment and misunderstanding. Listen to children, give them time, and wait for them to respond, as soon as they have developed sufficiently to do so. The young person who has been given time to organize his or her thoughts before expressing them is able to communicate with much more skill, than the one who has always had to compete for attention and fight to hold it.

Singing is pleasurable to the baby from birth, some would say even before. Rhythm is inborn, the first sounds during prenatal development are permeated by the mother's heart beat, a steady, measured, regular rhythm. These sounds of the mother's body system when recorded and played back have proved highly successful in calming crying babies. The tape and record may be acquired commercially.

Lullabies have always been sung to babies and children, and there is no reason why today's new generation should be deprived of such pleasures. Music is a common language and a vehicle of communication at any age. It is probably a more versatile vehicle than speech, and thus demands fair attention when considering the all round development of children. A mistake often made is that of exposing babies or children to a constant radio transmission. Many homes and nurseries work with a continuous background of 'pop' music. This prevents the child from hearing anything clearly, as he or she will not be able to select required sounds from the environment. This may well mean all that is heard is a jumble of meaningless noise, which could affect the development of language and understanding.

Bowel and bladder control

One of the biggest questions in the second year is that of bowel and bladder control, or *toilet training* as it was commonly called. Some mothers hold their tiny babies over a pot, there is no question of control, just knowing their habits of elimination, and pure luck. Of course it is desirable to have fewer soiled nappies, and to look forward to the time when they are not needed at all.

Control of the bowel and bladder will develop as the central nervous system matures. As with all aspects of maturation this is variable in different individuals, but has normally happened towards the end of the second year, to some degree. Most toddlers will be able to achieve control of their bowel function before their bladder control is refined and reliable. Girls tend to arrive at this stage earlier than boys. Some mothers claim that their children have become 'clean and dry' within a fortnight of taking the nappies off. This may well be true but often applies to the 2-year-old, who probably had been capable of control for some time.

It is worth starting to encourage the baby to experience the process of organized elimination towards the end of the first year. The tell-tale sign of a bowel movement becoming imminent are easily identifiable. The child will stop activity, become 'glassy eyed' and then begin to exert himself or herself. This is when a friendly suggestion regarding the pot may be made. Catching the moment develops into a cooperative programme of sociable toileting. The child prefers to be clean and dry, and enjoys the pleasure expressed by the adult. Movement is made easier without bulky nappies. There should be no display of distaste or anger when mistakes are made and obviously no punishments administered. Patience and encouragement are the key words as in all areas of learning, together with the shared joy of success and achievement.

It has often been said to a mother weary of nappy washing, 'Don't worry he won't go to school in nappies'. It is suprising how this possibility does seem a serious threat to mothers, even though reassurance is constant.

Being dry at night is the final hurdle in the process of total control of bowel and bladder. Some advocate 'lifting' of small children late at night, and if this causes no problems and the child does not wake up, then it will probably mean a few dry nights. Lifting is the disturbing of a child during a period of sleep to take him or her to the lavatory or pot. There seems to be little relationship between the amount of fluid drunk late in the evening, and a dry night. Therefore it is not a good idea to refuse fluid to a thirsty child with this in mind.

Without 'lifting' or reducing fluids, there will be dry nappies for the odd night at first, leading to a few together, with the occasional wet one. After a few dry nights the risk to leave the nappy off can be taken, protecting the bed with a waterproof sheet, and the baby in terry towelling trainers. If this is followed by a regular display of pleasure on finding each dry nappy, the chances are that the end is in sight. It must be remembered though that illness or any emotional stress can lead to accidents day or night. It may not be easy to identify the cause if it is an emotional one, because what will cause one child to react in this way, may well be totally ignored by another. In order to avoid carrying a 'potty' around when visiting, or on holiday, familiarize the child with the adult lavatory as soon as he or she can cope physically. There are special seats available and small platforms. Some children are frightened of the hole, by the flushing, and the disappearance of the contents. They may well justifiably fear a similar fate, if they were to fall in. This is quite logical and can be appreciated if the adult imagines a similar problem on a relative scale.

Last of all there is no set time limit when a child should be clean and dry, day and night, but if such control has not started to emerge by the end of the second year, there is no harm in seeking advice. As the child will normally communicate fairly well at this age, he or she ought to understand the idea unless there is something physically wrong. The development outlined applies to what is defined as normal.

Eating habits

Physical development will continue in a satisfactory way given that the child is well-nourished in all aspects, as well as the obvious one of feeding. Happy, secure, well-adjusted children will thrive better on the same diet than those who have to cope with problems such as insecurity. Such an emotion may temporarily emerge if a new baby arrives, the family move house, or even if a holiday is taken. One of the first signs of stress is often displayed through changes in habits of eating, whatever the age of the person, and small children soon realize the attention this can attract.

If the child refuses food, the best way is to remain relatively casual, at the same time noting how much has been consumed during the day. First eliminate or confirm the possibility of illness, offer extra fluids, probably containing added nourishment, such as beaten egg, and look for other causes. Accepting that the food rejected is normally popular with the child, it is usually sufficient to reinforce the child's position emotionally, by displaying affection rather more than usual, and avoiding absence of the mother or father figure, until the pattern of behaviour returns to normal. The short absence of a parent or the separation of the child for any reason at this stage causes a reaction similar to bereavement or total loss. The understanding of a period of time has not developed.

On the question of diet, this will be suitably mixed by the end of the second year, and attention should be paid to the fact that teeth and gums need regular exercise. Therefore foods which require chewing as well as biting need to be offered every day. It is surprising how few foods actually require any real effort to chew. Many children are very reluctant to make this effort.

At 2 years old physical movements will cover quite a range of identifiable skills: walking, running, anticipating obstacles, crouching, climbing, jumping and kicking are practised. Skipping comes much later, after hopping. In fact skipping is often difficult to perform even for a 4- to 5-year-old, girls usually mastering it first. Walking up and down stairs follows a developmental pattern and the 2-year-old will come down two feet at a time, to each step.

For much of the day this young child will be very active, adequate rest and sleep are essential. A rest will be welcome either late morning, or early afternoon, whichever suits both the child and the family. It does not matter whether the child always sleeps or not, but he or she does need the opportunity, whether outside in the pram, or in a cot. All children decide for themselves how long they will sleep, and ideally they will be happy and content to play quietly if sleep is not required.

Toys can be made available, and the environment inside or out, if chosen carefully, will provide sufficient to stimulate and interest the baby or child. Toys at this age are important but need not be expensive. Basically playthings should encourage use of the senses, and aid mobility. Opportunity to experiment is welcome and novelty is exciting. It is now that safety is of paramount importance as the 2-year-old has little sense or understanding of danger.

Danger is an area of awareness which develops according to the individual and there is a wide variation even between adults. Learning cannot be ensured here due to a programme of planned experience. The consequences of inappropriate action must be appreciated even feared, if the child is to learn beyond the basic sense of self-preservation. This instinct is insufficient protection in a modern technological world.

Toys should challenge without encouraging foolhardiness. The environment should provide a richness for experimentation and exploration within sensible limits. It is one of the most responsible tasks of those caring for young children that they guide them through the first years providing a balance between guidance and freedom.

Chapter 4
The Toddler Period

The toddler period may be defined as that between about 2 years and 4 years of age, although the baby/child actually toddles around much earlier than this.

The toddler represents a cocktail of child behaviour. He or she can be cooperative or antisocial, noisy or peaceful, hyperactive or reflective, happy one minute, and 'heart-broken' the next. The toddler though looking relaxed may be actively engaged in ignoring that cleaning up time has arrived (Fig. 4.1). The toddler is rarely bored or boring.

The period has been labelled 'the adolescence of childhood'. It certainly presents problems at times, just as adolescence seems to, and it is followed and preceded by a time when parents find their children particularly lovable and cooperative. This of course is a generalization and there are many exceptions, but it could be accepted that more behaviour problems emerge during these periods of development. As some of these problems are identified as characteristic of this stage, they will be looked at in detail.

CHARACTERISTIC BEHAVIOUR

Negativism

There is a time when it seems there is a programme of almost total non cooperation. A programme of severe testing of the patience and self control of the adult, who has hitherto been in a position of unapposed decision maker. Up to now the adult has, on the whole, displayed superiority, and has been able to distract or persuade a child who is disruptive. A new powerful word is quite suddenly acquired, together with an amazingly accurate sense of meaning. This of course is 'no'. It is used verbally and through body language. For example

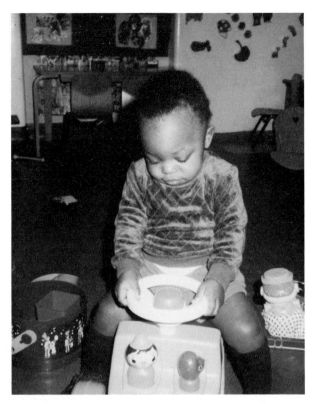

Fig. 4.1 A toddler at play.

it is a common picture to see a child who has been asked to 'come here' immediately 'going there'. They are totally precise in interpreting the opposite to that which is suggested at the time. It should be a simple solution to ask the child to perform in the opposite manner to that really hoped for, and consequently achieve the desired result. This does not work either, they seem to know in advance which behaviour will provoke the most entertaining reaction.

Unfortunately the answer is not a simple one, especially for the adult who does not know the child well. If the mother or father or other well known person is placed in a situation of conflict with a 2- to 3-year-old, there will be sufficient knowledge of each other to take the more hopeful line of action. The frustrating aspect is, what will solve the problem on one occasion, may well exacerbate it on another.

This stage will pass, it is a reflection of growing independence and a testing of this new urge to challenge the familiar, even attack it. The relative urge in adolescence often results in the young person rejecting the safe and familiar, by leaving home. It is seen by parents as total rejection, and for a time it may appear to be. It is sad if when the testing period has passed, which it surely will, reconciliation between the generations has become impossible.

Regression

A reversal to a former stage of development may be reflected physically, socially, emotionally or intellectually. It happens, to some extent, during illness at any stage in life due to the necessity to become once again dependent, in areas where independency has been achieved. Sometimes in the physical sense this is unavoidable, but is accepted and often enjoyed. It is the regression due to emotional stress, that may be observed during the third year.

New found skills such as bowel and bladder control, self feeding, and being happy without mother or father, are dispensed with, and the resulting pressures cause the adults to treat the child with a short measure of understanding. Both parties deserve sensitive attention. The parent honestly feels that the child is embarking on a deliberate programme of provocation, is selecting the appropriate areas for concentration, and hitting the most vulnerable spot every time. The child feels that love is being withdrawn unfairly, especially if the cause of the trouble is a new baby. After all, the baby does all these things, and still seems to be receiving all the attention, hitherto his or her own, and not shared with anyone. It seems reasonable that if he or she behaves like a baby, all will be as it used to be. When this does not happen the older child becomes totally bewildered, and the behaviour probably even more confused. These children need to 'find themselves' again, and will need special attention, and time, without the baby, to establish their real position once more. Emphasis could be placed on the things that they, and not the baby can do, relating them to being grown-up, more like mummy and daddy or a favourite mature relative. Helping with the baby is popular, but it is not a good idea to leave them alone together. Jealousy is a very powerful emotion in human terms at any age. If the mother has been away from her child for some reason, even for a day or two, similar regressive behaviour may emerge.

Tantrums

The 2- to 3-year-old is invariably labelled as a prima donna of temper tantrums. These can range from angry crying with throwing of objects, to self inflicted pain, such as biting, head banging, or breath holding.

The most familiar type of behaviour is the screaming child. These children throw themselves to the ground, kicking wildly, seeming out of control, and yet capable of stopping and recommencing with amazing dramatic expertise. The child who is deeply unhappy, or in pain, cannot display this control. There is no suggestion that a temper tantrum is a happy affair, but it requires different handling. Once again it is a normal stage of development, however irritating and embarrassing at the time.

There is usually a cause for this eruption, and very often it happens when the child either wants something, or wants to do something that the adult will not allow at the time. It may be that 'something' has been given or allowed under different circumstances, and the child can be forgiven for not appreciating that most adults are inconsistent. Sadly though, this is true, and is reflected in their handling of children in many cases. For instance, why can the child walk sometimes, and at other times when mother is in a hurry, have to ride in the push chair? Why should the child walk quickly sometimes, and yet be content to stand patiently, either in a queue, or whilst mother chats for 20 minutes to a friend? Why can't the pudding be before the dinner, the child would like it better that way round? The list of illogical habits of adults is a very long one, when you are 2½ years old.

Sleeping

Another basic function vital to a healthy well-being, yet apparently the cause of many problems is sleep. The general idea tends to prevail that 'good' babies and children sleep according to what is convenient for their elders, and that 'naughty' or 'difficult' babies and children do the opposite.

All babies and children are as unique as their elders and their needs vary. They do not stay awake because it is more enjoyable, although this will at times obviously be the case. They often are simply not ready to sleep, either because they are not tired, have had too much recent stimulation, or are, quite simply, afraid to lose consciousness. For instance, if a parent or other loved one has disappeared, even temporarily, the anxiety caused can be traumatic. As has already been pointed out, it is similar to the shock of bereavement. Consequently, to sleep means losing control, as the child is unable to keep watch on the remaining adult or adults. This may happen after moving house or when on holiday, the child feels the need to check constantly on that which is familiar, and represents security, in his or her world. This can lead to frequent awakenings during the night. What is required is reassurance not an irritable response from a weary adult. This is easy to recommend, but very difficult to carry out, when the real situation presents itself. It is worthwhile remembering this as the insensitive, but understandable, anger only causes everyone to have a prolonged battle in the middle of the night.

There will probably be attendant rituals at bedtime, established very early and thereafter rigidly adhered to. Altering these can cause upsets, so try to remember order and process, especially if other things have been changed. If lights are usually left on somewhere, then do not suddenly decide that it is time to economize in the middle of winter when it is very dark. After the long light evenings of summer, the gradual darkening will probably be accepted.

If particular toys are taken to bed, or a music box is left on, or stories read, such habits can continue happily into late childhood. Music may be welcome at bedtime, and reading a story or having one read still rounds off the day satisfactorily. If a habit of companionship before sleeping is established, it can present an opportunity to talk about problems, worries, joys and successes, an opportunity which is almost vital in late childhood and adolescence.

The bed or bedroom should never be linked to a threat or punishment. It should be a peaceful, happy place where the child goes to enjoy one of the most pleasurable activities, that of untroubled sleep. This is in the real sense an activity, the body is busy repairing and refreshing itself in preparation for another busy period. The mind is given some 'time off' although of course it continues to operate as indicated through dreams. It has been said that some individuals may remember information played during a period of sleep. If this system worked efficiently for everyone the whole education system could be altered.

When children are unable to sleep during the traditional hours, they should be free to play safely in their cots. The problem becomes more complex when they are old enough to be in a bed, and could come to some harm if left free to wander about during the night. In this situation, a harness, although it does appear restrictive, may give everyone more peace of mind, especially for a child whose sense of danger, and of self preservation is slow to develop. All parents have at some time taken their babies or children into their own beds. Some experts recommend it, others strongly forbid such practice. It can be dangerous if the father is there; mothers seem to have an instinctive sense, which prevents them from rolling over onto their babies. Later, although both mother and child may enjoy the experience it is best kept to a special time or ritual, otherwise the child will not appreciate the variation in such allowances. Adults must be seen to be consistent. One such 'special' time could be Sunday morning, or any other, when members of the family do not have to leave the house for work or school. Father may be persuaded to bring a cup of tea to his family whilst they enjoy the luxury together with a chance to be close to each other. Those who point out the risks of such escapades are correct, but if common sense prevails the pleasure is worth taking with reasonable precautions.

Aggression

Emotions may be displayed in a variety of ways and this applies to aggression. It can be directed at other people, inanimate objects or at self with self inflicted pain. If all adults freely expressed their emotions they would probably indulge in very similar behaviour patterns, as do children of 2-3 years of age.

Normally the stage of violent behaviour passes. Those who unfortunately fail to develop sufficiently to leave such a stage behind, frequently become involved in situations which demand a control which is beyond their personal boundary. Once again the adolescent years reflect such problems of physical control, when under emotional stress. At the same time it should be recognized that physical exertion can, and does, offer a vehicle for emotional release. If a safe and socially acceptable vehicle is chosen it can be labelled therapeutic. Examples such as chopping wood, making bread, cleaning out a room, have been offered as useful vehicles. Anger which is refused expression may be potentially much more dangerous than that which is accepted as reasonable. It can build up, as incidents occur, and result in a serious violent outburst, when one small irritation becomes 'the straw' breaking the camel's back.

Therefore, children should be allowed their anger, they need to be guided into ways of expressing this powerful emotion, and they need to learn when it is justified and when it is not acceptable. Society has need of those who are capable of being justifiably angry, capable of channelling their energy into avenues which are purposeful, and capable of changing that which has given rise to the justifiable anger.

Elizabeth Fry was angry when she discovered the conditions under which female prisoners and their children were forced to exist. Conservationists are angry when they see the beauty and innocence of flora and fauna being sacrificed. It is this sort of anger that when transformed into purposeful action, has caused changes which will go down in the history of society and ecology. Children must learn that anger can be good, they need to experience and master the emotion.

Habits

Thumb and finger sucking are very familiar habits and it is difficult to advise on how, when, or if, to make some effort to prevent this. Most children will naturally stop sucking when they mature sufficiently not to need this comfort. There could be some relationship though, between this very early habit and the later ones of smoking cigarettes and pipes, and biting nails. They all offer oral satisfaction which reflects a basic instinctive need. It may also reflect basic insecurity, but such statements are obviously subjective and depend very much on individual points of view.

Finger and thumb sucking over a long period can cause teeth to become displaced, and specialized treatment may be required to correct this. Some mothers tend to offer comfort orally, e.g. with sweets, dummies, dinky feeders whenever a baby or child is upset. Naturally this establishes a habit and becomes the norm, lasting throughout life. As has been mentioned before, too many adults seek comfort in food, sweets, drinks and smoking. These palliatives simply mask the real problem, and do not even begin to present any solutions.

The sweetness in the dinky feeder simply becomes the box of chocolates for the adult. Those who care for young children are responsible for many of the harmful habits they develop later in life.

Busy, happy, stable children will hopefully not need the extra self induced comfort of sucking for much longer than their toddler period. If it does continue, however, it is useless to draw attention to it constantly and nag. Make the children's world as secure as possible, and make sure that they have plenty to keep them busy during their waking hours. Remember, very few teenagers suck their thumbs, and the one or two who do, seem to be perfectly well-adjusted, as a rule.

Use of imagination

Young children often create imaginary people, animals, or other beings for themselves, and although there probably is a good reason, there is usually nothing to worry about. Once again it is an appropriate behaviour pattern which occurs in early childhood, and disappears quite suddenly. Fears and unasked questions may be projected through the imaginary being. For example a child may ask for a light to be left on 'Because Benson likes the light' or 'Benson is afraid of the dark'. Blame may be laid on Benson 'He broke the plate, isn't he clumsy?' or 'I can't eat my dinner, Benson wants it'. It is not fair at this stage to force the child into the situation of admitting that the 'being' does not exist. After all, he or she is probably encouraged to believe in other imaginary beings through stories that adults tell, and certainly is persuaded that 'Father Christmas' is a good idea. It may be the foundation for future faith in something which cannot necessarily be seen, and the growth of faith is a delicate and very precious attribute which is simply too important to tamper with. At this age or stage of development in terms of relative understanding, the story of Christmas will be close to any other such as 'Goldilocks' or 'Cinderella'. It would be interesting to record at which age imaginary beings normally disappear, and at which age religious faith could be said to emerge. The intangible nature of such phenomena obviously causes such findings to be almost impossible to achieve.

Whether imaginary beings are used as scapegoats or for company does not really matter, as long as their importance fades as the child reaches the age of reason, commonly accepted as about 7 years of age. It has already been established that rates of development vary considerably, and obviously nothing magic happens overnight on the seventh birthday, so this must always be taken into consideration especially when looking at emotional changes.

Masturbation

As babies learn about their body, they play with their hands and feet quite happily, moving them about provides much amusement. This is accepted by the mother as a very attractive picture is presented. When, however, babies handle their genitals, some mothers immediately show concern. This activity is natural and is simply part of getting to know their own bodies. They find that certain places when fondled offer a new pleasure and satisfaction, so obviously this activity is repeated whenever the opportunity arises, and when they feel the need for such comfort.

If the habit worries the adult it is a good idea to distract the child, give him or her something interesting to do, to keep his or her hands busy. Avoid drawing attention to the activity which is causing the problem. In fact masturbation is practised by many normal adults, male and female, throughout life. What has to be learned is, that in this society it is unacceptable behaviour in public, or in company.

Great care should be taken that adult reaction does not indicate that there is anything 'dirty' or 'wicked' about masturbation. Also, that old wives tales, such as, 'It will make you blind' are not allowed to be voiced even jokingly to the child.

Those who inappropriately deal with behaviour involving 'toilet training' and masturbation when caring for young children may be responsible for adolescent and adult problems regarding sexuality, attitudes to nudity, and other personal aspects of life.

Chapter 5
The Preschool and Early School Child

PHYSICAL AND INTELLECTUAL DEVELOPMENT

Between the ages of approximately 3 and 8 years, much observable growth takes place. Alongside the physical development of the skeletal and muscular system, there is a parallel emergence of skills, associated with such a complex machine. In order that such skills develop smoothly, intellectual functioning matures at an accompanying though variable rate. This means it must never be assumed that a child of any particular physical size necessarily reflects matching intellectual behaviour.

Nature seems to programme intense physical growth, whilst allowing mental growth to 'take it easy'. This happens in reverse. For example, the growth spurt in adolescence is often accompanied by immature or regressive behaviour. It seems unfortunate that boys and girls encounter important examinations at the same chronological age, when it is accepted that they mature at different rates. Girls tend to approach life more seriously at an earlier age, and tend to perform better academically at 16 years of age, although boys catch up within a year or two. These are established trends and must not be used as definitive arguments in specific situations.

Between 3 and 8 years, there is a period of relative stability. On the whole children cause their parents and teachers little anxiety. The frustrations of the toddler period and the emerging of self identity have been largely resolved. They are open to reason, especially if they have had the benefit of consistent handling and they 'see' their place within a family unit. So much is demanded of the children socially and intellectually during this period, that the calmness is particularly appropriate.

The learning phase

During the 3- to 8-year-old stage, children will learn to be socially independent, leaving their parents for short periods, and find their place in school communities. They will learn to make certain decisions within that environment and learn to communicate, in an appropriate way, with people other than the immediate family. They will learn to test their bodies, to make demands upon their bodies, and to gain pleasure and confidence in acquiring physical skills. They will be able to communicate through the written word, and will be introduced to concepts of number, weight, volume, distance, and time. The environment, the world, and the basic laws which govern them will also be covered. They will learn to express emotions, to laugh and to cry, when and where it is acceptable and/or socially appropriate. This list is by no means exhaustive, but is undoubtably impressive.

Development profiles

To illustrate the progress outlined it will be useful to look at profiles of children at one year intervals. Such profiles will almost certainly fail to reflect in total any other particular child of a similar age, thus emphasizing the variables which occur. They are however more helpful for many readers, than the familiar progress charts of expected behaviour. Such a guide would tend to detract from the character profile, as well as serve as a possible irritant within the text. As you read them, try to identify which area of development is being referred to.

MARK IS THREE

Mark is just 3 years old, and well and truly demonstrating his instinctive urge to explore and experiment. A good command of his body movements helps here, and a fairly reliable knowledge of his own limitations, offers a reasonable guide to safety and self preservation.

The physical rate of growth has slowed down, although Mark

has gained roughly 10 cm (4 inches) in the last 12 months, and he weighs 14 kg (32 lbs). He is larger than most of his girlfriends of the same age, and moves in a child's, rather than a toddler's, fashion. Mark goes up and down stairs with confidence, although often he prefers to descend by placing both feet on each step, then jumping the last two! He can control his speed of movement, also his direction. He likes to walk along walls, climb obstacles, stand on one leg, and particularly enjoys the extra speed offered by a pedal car or tricycle. Mark likes to be watched and admired, and will perform acrobatic feats for an appreciative audience.

There is already evidence of a striving for perfection, and like other 3-year-olds, he will insist on doing something over and over again, until satisfied. As already suggested, accompanying this smoother physical development, a more defined intellectual growth can be diagnosed. Periods of concentration are more extended, and toys and playthings should, at this age, allow for such activity. Jig-saws and other puzzles, construction kits, play people, drawing materials and modelling materials, all serve to encourage periods of concentrated effort, linked to expression and imagination. Solving puzzles, at times, is by trial and error rather than visual interpreta-tion. This is illustrated by the approach to the familiar 'posting box' puzzle, when all the shapes may be tried at random, until they fit the appropriate hole.

Although the concepts of vertical and horizontal have been dis-played in brick building and drawing, it is interesting to observe the reaction to requests to fold paper diagonally, or copy shapes such as triangles or diamonds.

Language development is advancing at a rapid rate, and Mark has been fortunate enough to have parents, relatives and friends who communicate with him avoiding any tendency to 'baby language'. It should be remembered that, at all ages human beings understand more than they have the ability to express. Mark needs to hear new words regularly, in order to incorporate them accurately into his own vocabulary. He understands about 1,000 different words, which is quite an amazing achievement in such a short time. Some-times he will mispronounce, or adapt a word which he cannot man-age to pronounce properly, but needs and wishes to use. For example, music is 'umix'. Although some of these words are attractive, even amusing, it is advisable not to display such amusement, too often, otherwise one of two things may occur. Firstly he may tend to avoid using new words or attempting more complicated ones for fear of being laughed at. Secondly he may continue to use pet expressions when proper pronunciation is easily manageable. There are some adults whose children having grown through the age of language experimentation, still continue to use pet names and expressions. It is embarrassing to hear such phrases as 'I must go and wash my paws', 'Where is my neckie' (napkin). In the same way, names lovingly given in early childhood are best kept there—Didikins (David) does not suit a middle aged man, neither does Christopher Dick!

Mark knows his name and is aware of his sex. He is beginning to use prepositions appropriately, illustrated by using a model room or another layout, and following instructions on its arrangement. The amusing habit of talking himself through an activity continues, since it commenced a few months ago. The monologue, however, is much more intelligible, although reality and imagination are beautifully and conveniently woven together.

Mark is already at the stage where he will learn by rote for the pleasure of recitation. He not only knows nursery rhymes, but also a few short poems. He is very familiar with the sequence of some of his favourite stories, and will be quick to interrupt if the adult tries to miss a page, or make up part of the story to speed things along.

Music has always been part of Mark's life. Not the constant background of 'pop' music, but records, along with popular radio music at certain times. He has developed a love of military marches and some of the stirring songs presented by organisations such as the Salvation Army. He usually moves around to records, but in contrast welcomes the opportunity to listen quietly to a story tape or record, or join in one of the children's song or rhyme records.

Accompanying this obvious skill of learning and remembering, which needs to be encouraged and nourished, is his own method of adding to his fund of knowledge by regular questioning of 'Who?', 'Where?' and 'What?'. Such questions are often asked at an inappropriate moment, but Mark is lucky enough to be able to expect some sort of constructive or helpful response in most instances. The simple prefix of 'what' or 'where' can present a problem to the adult whose best solution is to admit ignorance and suggest a joint effort to find out, if necessary at a future appointed date, e.g. 'Later on, when I have put the washing out!' It is almost dangerous to the emerging intellect to constantly 'block off' questions, which will naturally be asked. The child will learn in a negative way, that it is not worth asking, and the urge to know will be supressed.

Independence in personal areas is developing well, and Mark can manage to eat and drink with a fair degree of social competence as well as natural efficiency. Such development is fostered in the nursery setting where children are able to lay tables, serve food and generally socialise between themselves without too much interference from adults (Fig. 5.1). Mark uses a fork and spoon, rather than a knife and fork, the latter demanding a complex skill. He obviously has likes and dislikes, but allowing for these, his diet is similar to that of his parents, and thus adequate and well-balanced. All children like small snacks sometimes, and Mark's mother has encouraged him to develop the habit of enjoying fruit, fresh or dried, nuts, nut

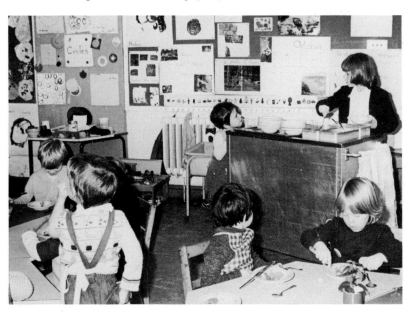

Fig. 5.1 Social skills such as laying tables and serving food can be fun to learn.

bars, a handful of dry cereal or a piece of flapjack at such times. Obviously on occasions he will have an ice-cream, chocolate biscuit or sweet. Such pleasures have their important place in life, at any age!

Mark can undress himself with relative ease, it is the reverse procedure which presents some problems. Back and front still seem to reposition themselves with frustrating regularity, as do the left and right of shoes and Wellington boots. Most of the time it really does not matter to the child, it is the adults who require these things to be correct. Shoes on the wrong foot will cause no problems for a short time. When Mark looks at a coat or jacket and sees the front, he is unable to manipulate visually, that if he approaches it, the front will end up on his own back. Some children have been observed going through this procedure time and time again, with disbelief a forerunner to frustration. One of the most amusing was a small child with a balaclava helmet, whose reasoning appeared to him logical, but he finished up three or four times with the hole for his face at the back of his head. Each time the garment came off, and each time he obviously could not believe what happened. Eventually his mother simply 'swivelled' it round, a visual interpretation not yet developed in the child.

Mark is proud of his control over his bowel and bladder functioning, although the former has been reliably established for well over a year now. Only if he is unwell will there be any doubt about his efficiency in this area. On the other hand, he will still avoid going to empty his bladder, if he is particularly engrossed in an interesting activity. It is not to be expected that Mark will always be able to clean himself satisfactorily after using the toilet, but this presents no real problem. He decides whether or not help is acceptable, according to the mood of the moment. Washing his hands needs a reminder, and drying them is more often than not fairly haphazard. Watch an adult, or take particular notice next time you use a handtowel, to appreciate the complexity of the skill.

One of the most interesting characteristics of Mark's play pattern is the obvious awareness of other children as companions, rather than other isolated individuals engaged upon a similar activity. He will join others and play in a cooperative way for a period of time, then revert to solitary or parallel play (Fig. 5.2), or change groups quite spontaneously. As a result of this new awareness of the value of companionship, he has experienced and understood the necessity for 'taking turns', and waiting for a share of a special toy. Mark also seeks support and help from adults, rather than strongly refusing to accept such aid, as he tended to do, at the age of 2. He will also listen to a verbal interpretation of problem solving, and make attempts to convert this into physical manipulation. This illustrates the emerging concepts of spatial relationships, and transfer of such concepts into appropriate action.

Mark also understands that there are times when he obeys without question, such as during outings, in areas where traffic is a hazard. It is particularly important that all children know, through the consistent and stable relationship developed with the adults in their lives, when it is vital to respond directly. One child dashed into the road, and his mother instructed him to stay on the centre island. She did not suggest or persuade, but gave a clear command. She herself

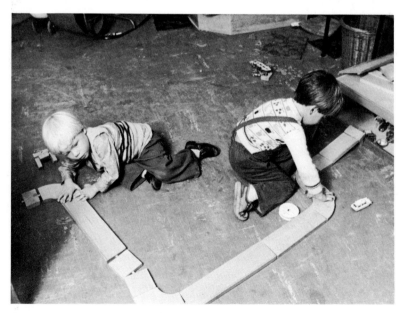

Fig. 5.2 Parallel play involves children playing alongside each other with the same toy and yet seemingly independent of each other.

made no attempt to pursue the child knowing that he was already frightened and isolated, surrounded by strangers and moving traffic. She then waited for a safe moment and walked at a normal pace to collect her child. This took a cool nerve and total trust on both sides.

At 3 years children are still a mixture of emotions. They will alternate from the happy, loving and sociable beings, to the angry uncooperative and unreasonable ones. What they need is the constant support to enable them to handle these changes, which occur not of choice, but rather as a controlling influence. They always need an acceptable avenue offered back into the happy loving atmosphere which sometimes seems to elude them. These situations have a strong relationship with emotions in adolescence.

Mark is about to experience the arrival of a new baby sister or brother, and in common with many young children of his age, he will almost certainly have to overcome and accommodate initial feelings of uncertainty. Everything seems to indicate, that his adaption to the new situation will be smooth.

JENNY IS FOUR

Jenny is 4 years old, and she herself will 'talk' about her capabilities and feelings. (This has been translated into mature language.)

'I have grown quite appreciably since I had my third birthday, although I am not quite as tall and heavy as most of the boys at my age. I have grown about 7.5 cm (3 inches), and gained a couple of kilograms, which seems very little compared with my record during my first year of life.

I enjoy running, hopping, and skipping around; the boys find skipping quite difficult, and we all laugh at nursery school when they try. They do not seem to mind, and even make it funnier for us, so we laugh even more. Maybe they really could do it if they tried, but they enjoy the laughing more. I like nursery school, where I can play with lots of people, and choose from lots of different things to do. At first I would have liked Mummy to stay, but she did promise to come back, after looking at all the things I was going to do, and she always keeps her promises. Otherwise she will explain that it is not fair to make them. The times when I would like her or Daddy there,

are when I am hurt, or I do not feel well, or when I have made something special, and I want to show them straight away. I like to play
with the boys and girls, although the boys get very rough and noisy
at times, and even mess up the games for the other children. The
teachers try to prevent this, but the boys will act suddenly, and then
will even help to repair what they have destroyed. I do not think they
can help it sometimes.

When we play in the Home Corner, only 4 children are allowed
in at the same time. The boys like to be 'Daddy' and go to work.
They like being the 'baby' too, but either way, we girls tend to be
the bosses, and the boys do as we tell them, or we do not always let
them play. In any case they always have to ask to play, and if we like
them, we will probably tell someone else to go out of the game. We
have to keep to 4 you see. We usually dress up in different clothes to
start playing in the Home Corner, and then if we like we can often
keep the clothes on for a long time, even though we are doing other
things. It makes me feel special. We must take them off if we go out
to ride bicycles or play on the climbing frames or swings. I cannot
remember why.

I like drawing and writing, and I can find my name on the milk
bottle. I can copy writing on my pictures, and 'do' my name,
because mine is not too difficult. Some of the children have such difficult names, even my teacher cannot pronounce or spell them easily. They have to ask their Mummies or Daddies.

We even cook and sew at school, and the boys are good just like
Daddy. He can cook, and is very good at using the sewing machine,
Mummy says he is better than she is. I do not think she is very keen
at sewing, she likes gardening better, and I help her as well as having my own special garden. I just wish I did not have to wait so long
for seeds to grow, it seems like forever when Mummy says how
many weeks it will be before I have flowers. One day I seemed to
have waited for those weeks, so I dug the seeds up to see how they
were getting along, and then they never did grow at all! I wonder
why they stopped when I looked at them. I just keep on growing
anyway. So do trees and things, and people are looking at them all
the time. I wonder why things like Teddy Bears and cars do not
grow, that would be great fun. Things like that do happen in stories.

I have favourite colours, I know which is which, but I like to change my favourite, sometimes every day. I like asking lots of questions, and know that the best answers come from 'Why?' and 'How?'. Sometimes I already know the answers, but that makes me feel even better, when my teacher agrees with what I already thought. It gives me some of her time too, and that can be very difficult to obtain. We do have the opportunity to tell the rest of the group about our 'news', but the problems are, that in the first place I do not want to hear everyone else's, and also I have to wait so long. I need to keep going over my news in my own mind, in order to be ready, that I cannot listen properly. And then, my teacher does not have time to ask everyone, and she suddenly stops and I feel cross and disappointed. When I am bigger I can write it all down.

I like helping people. At school we have special jobs, and at home I help Mummy and Daddy. Grandma and Grandpa let me help too, and I can often do more special things for them, because they do not have to hurry so much. Grandma is going to teach me to crochet when I am bigger, which is something she tried to teach Mummy when she was a little girl. She does 'tatting' too and not many grown-ups can do that. It is very nice being with Grandma, but sometimes she goes to sleep in the afternoons, and I have to be quiet and not disturb her.

I used to go to sleep during the day, but I'm much too big now. I do not really like going to bed at all, because I'm usually much too busy. I do have some favourite 'people' to talk to, and I can usually hear noises from downstairs, but if it is very dark, I like to have the light on in the landing, then everything still looks familiar. When we went on holiday I did not go to sleep quickly, and I woke up in the night not knowing where I was. This did frighten me. Being lost is very frightening indeed. I remember losing Mummy in the supermarket recently, and I thought I had found her, only to look up from a familiar pair of denim trousers, to a strange face. I tried to be grown-up, but I soon began to cry, and a kind adult lifted me high enough to find her face. It is very difficult to be on the same level as lots and lots of similar lower halves of people. Normally I do sleep all night, but I like getting up when I wake and this is sometimes rather too early for my parents. I cannot tell the time yet, so I do not know.

Sometimes I creep in beside my parents. This is a treat, because Mummy has a cup of tea in bed at the weekends, and then I have one too. I have a special cuddle too, and we talk about things without hurrying. My baby brother is too small to share this time with us, but he sometimes wakes in the night, because his tummy is too small to last until morning. He may need his nappy changing too.

I am glad that I am so grown-up, and can help Mummy at home. I fetch and carry things for her, and do small jobs like laying the table, and reminding her when it starts to rain and the washing is on the line. The baby cannot do anything like this, but we all love him and talk to him a lot, because he knows we are his family. When he first arrived he seemed to get in the way, and I sometimes wished we could send him back. Before, my parents could listen or help me, without the baby needing them first. But we still manage lots of time when he is asleep, and he has his turn while I am at Nursery School. It was lucky, that when I started there, the baby had not arrived, otherwise Mummy might not have been able to stay as she did, for the first couple of days, and if I had needed her, she may just have been too busy attending to him.

Fortunately, I am also big enough to dress myself, apart from tying bows and doing back fastenings. My Mummy makes sure that when I go to school I am wearing 'easy' clothes and shoes. Some poor children have a lot of trouble if they are in a hurry to use the toilet, and others take ages to change for the paddling pool, and to get dressed afterwards. They have to queue up for help. All my things have my name on too, and I do not have to worry too much about losing something. It is nice to hear the teacher say 'What a sensible Mother you have Jenny'. My Mummy is better than anybody else's, I know that, but when the teacher says such things, it makes me feel very proud.

I do have some special friends, and they come to play at my house. Sometimes we play together, and sometimes I play with one thing, and my friend will do something different, but we still talk about what we are doing. I like making a milkshake for us, and asking my friends to choose their flavour. I like going to other people's houses, but I like mine the best.

Soon I will go to the 'big school', and that is where I will learn to read and write properly and do 'real work'. I am looking forward to that, as I will be able to read stories to my baby brother. I want to do all this quickly, because I am very impatient for things to happen.'

The five-year-old

Physically, the 5-year-old presents an attractive, well-coordinated young human frame, approximately two thirds of his or her potential height, thus allowing for some prediction of eventual height to be assessed. Growth spurts have given way to the smoother, slower physical development characteristic of the next few years. In contrast, intellectual functioning, given the stimulation and opportunity, takes off at an accelerated rate. Refined body control accompanies this mental development and enables acquired skills to be expressed and observed. The 5-year-old will hold a painting, drawing, or writing tool in such a way as to achieve a fine degree of control. Learning new skills seems to dominate other purposes in life.

Five is an age where life should be without problems, as the profile of the 5-year-old will demonstrate.

MARY IS FIVE

Mary is 5 and her urge to learn is constantly seeking new boundaries. She can swim with confidence and enjoyment, her father having taught her. Or rather, her father took her with him to the pool, or into the sea from the age of a few months. Mary quite simply put to good use her inherited skill to survive in the natural environment. Nobody ever told her how to breathe under water, or had to persuade her to enjoy her face covered in water. It is the confidence and courage of the parents that is put to the test in introducing very young children to water. It should never be necessary for them to experience the panic of fear in order to learn to swim.

As Mary has older brothers and sisters, she is always exposed to models which are more skilful than she is. They present to her a wide range of abilities, and therefore she is well on the way to becoming adept in many areas. One sister is musically inclined, and Mary is already singing in tune, and picking out notes on the xylophone. A brother is keen on sport, therefore various outgrown tools of sport are available for Mary to practise with, without first showing the inclination or preference. The whole family are keen on walking, so all the children are familiar with their natural environment. They can all name some of the trees, insects and flowers which many children never know. They appreciate what happens in the country as the seasons change.

Apart from the formal learning within the school programme, it is not difficult to appreciate how the children of such family units are distinctly advantaged. It has little to do with money or social class, although this is the excuse often given. It has everything to do with attitudes and good, responsible parenting.

Mary handles her world with a sense of immediacy, and basic single relationships. She can compare, arrange in order, and argue the reason for a phenomena. Multiple relationships, however, present a problem, as do abstract concepts. For example, the side view of a person or animal may well have two visible eyes, when drawn by a 5-year-old, just as a similar view of a vehicle may well show four wheels in a row. The child draws what is known, rather than what a 7-year-old will appreciate cannot be seen from a particular angle. Related to this is the difficulty encountered by 5-year-olds in putting themselves mentally, in another physical position. Set up a situation, e.g. with dolls, action men, and ask a 5-year-old if a specific doll would be able to 'see' a specific other. Do it with the children themselves and allow them to confirm or otherwise, whether their concept was correct. A quick tip related to this idea is for adults when planning any area for children—kneel down, consider the views, and decide whether or not the environment is arranged intelligently with the children literally in mind.

To illustrate the single/multi-relationship concept, take a set of logic blocks with different colours, shapes and thicknesses. First of all ensure that the children understand the names and adjectives you intend to use, as you are testing, not the vocabulary, but the concept. Make sure that they can all see. Then ask the children to find something:

a   exactly the same,
b   one thing different,

c two things different,
d three things different.
It may be necessary to present an example each time. Some 5-year-olds are able to do this, but it should not automatically be expected of them.

Mary understands that groups of objects with similar characteristics are given names, such as flowers, sweets or people. She also understands what a daffodil is, a chocolate, and an old man. What she is unable to comprehend is the direct relationship between the two, without need for confusion. Presented with four daffodils and three daisies, she will probably agree, that there are more daffodils than daisies, but not be able to decide whether there are more daffodils or more flowers.

In a similar way, an equal number of items placed in a row spaced out, will almost always be 'more', than the same number set in a pile. Conservation of number is not firmly established. At the same stage of development the child will not fully appreciate other properties remain constant. For example, a metre rule is placed alongside another, their ends parallel. The child will say they are the 'same'. Push one forward so it appears longer at one end, and the child will probably say, it is now in fact longer than the other.

As well as accepting the rules of sharing, and taking turns, Mary is able to apply basic rules to competitive activities, and the social art of losing has its foundation around this age. Playing card and board games at home does help, and sensible parents do not allow children to win, more than is kind and natural. Other children will not make any allowances at all. They all meet others who are better than they are at many things and at which they may have thought they were superior. It is a hard lesson to learn, that on some the gifts appear to have been showered in plenty, whereas others have to work extremely hard to achieve similar successes.

Right and wrong, to Mary, depends entirely on the degree of the misdemeanour or the result, not on the intention. To break three things, is worse than one, even though the former was an accident and the latter intentional.

The 5-year-old will usually be responsible and competent enough to play beyond the confines of the garden depending on the immedi-

ate home environment. For some, this would obviously be impossible. Depending on this criterion, Mary could go to a shop and buy a
single item, or a couple if a note is written. She could take a short
message or visit a neighbour round the corner, avoiding crossing
any road. Having said this, it is appreciated how threatening the
present day environment is, and judgement must rest with the responsible adult. The purpose of stating the capability, is to illustrate the
developmental stage, not to recommend any particular activity.

During the first few months at school Mary caught chicken-pox.
She was more upset about missing school than anything else, and
her attack was a mild one. It is very difficult to resist scratching the
spots, and those in her hair were particularly irritating. Now she
displays the sites of one or two spots like battle wounds, and with the
accompanying air of the resigned experience of the victim. It is to be
hoped that she does not grow into one of those individuals who relish
relating gruesome histories of illnesses and operations!

Mary's greatest achievement is the skill of reading. She has mastered the basic procedures of left to right, and phonetic recognition,
together with some whole word recognition. This means that she can
make some attempt at any new word, and is even realizing, that
'breaking down', and 'building up' again, can achieve success.
Breaking down involves taking a word and reducing it into smaller
units, then building these units into the whole word again, e.g.
carpenter, car—pen—ter.

In Mary's bedroom there is a wide selection of books, and she
spends time 'reading' them. When the book is too advanced, she will
quite happily make up her own story from the pictures. What is
important is the fact that already books are her friends, and in the
future will become a source of pleasure, challenge and information.
Girls often acquire the skill of reading with more ease than boys, and
Mary is no exception. There is no firm guide as to when a child
should begin to read. It is not a natural skill, but one which must be
learned. If any child reaches the age of 7 without showing the ability
to start reading, it is fair to that child to seek help and advice, assum-
ing that he or she has been afforded all the stimulation and guidance
one would expect in the normal school situation. Mary is a happy,
well-adjusted child.

ROBERT IS SIX. ROBERT READS HIS DIARY

7.30   I was woken up by Mummy opening the curtains, and telling me that the sun was shining. First of all I looked under the pillow to see if there was a 20 pence piece there, instead of my beautiful tooth. Until they started to come out I had twenty, now I have eighteen, and just appearing, the wavy edge of my first grown-up tooth. It was lucky that no-one was using the toilet, I cannot wait long in the morning. I checked the army under the bed, they guard me during the night, in case the Daleks come. I dressed myself well, although my shirt tails usually hang out! I do not wear a tie for school, because I cannot do it myself yet. As it is the summer I wear sandals, and I can fasten those.

8.00   Mummy sits with my brother and me for breakfast, but she does not have her's until we have gone to school. She says she needs that bit of peace and quiet, after the morning rush. I suppose part of the trouble is, that I suddenly remember what I need for school just at the last moment. I know this is difficult, but I honestly do forget, until I am thinking about school in the morning. Often it is not terribly important but if we have a colour table or nature corner, I like to put something on it.

8.30   We all walk to my school, where my elder brother leaves to go to his part for Juniors. I will go there when I am seven. On the way we usually meet some friends, and the Mothers talk together. We like to get to school in time to play outside for a while, then we can organize our gangs for the day. As some of the boys are much bigger than the smallest ones, even though we are all roughly the same age, it is a good idea to have some of them in our gang. In fact the smallest boy on our graph measured 96 cm and Roger, the biggest was 142 cm. He says he is going to be a policeman like his uncle. We went to the Police Station when they had an Open Day, and some of the policemen are quite small compared with Roger's uncle. We asked them how tall they were and made a graph like the one showing our own heights.

9.00 We went into school for assembly, and the headmaster talked about helping our parents in the holidays. I listened for a bit, then I showed my friend one of my soldiers. I usually take something to school to show the others, and we make a game with what we bring. We like playing wars and fighting, I like being dead, but it gets boring, so we come alive again very quickly.

9.20 In the morning we work in our writing or number books, and sometimes we read to the teacher, or one of the ladies who come in to help her. It is quicker to go to the ladies or the big girls, because they help us a bit more. Then we can have our cards marked, and say we have done it. Reading is a nuisance, and the girls are always ahead of me, but it really doesn't matter because my models are better than theirs. I wrote some news and drew a picture in my book. If I need a new word, I have to wait in a queue for my teacher to write it, so I try to think of words I know. Sometimes I wait for a long time and then I find that the word was in my dictionary, but I did not look properly.

10.15 We went outside to play and I had a very good battle with aeroplanes and bombs. Whilst I was being a bomber jet, I knocked two girls over with my 'wings'. The teacher was cross, but you have to go round very fast in a war, or the enemy can intercept. I got a bit dirty at playtime, but I rubbed it off.

10.30 Then we played with money, and the supermarket corner. We can buy two things, and take turns at being the cashier. I did some proper sums in my work book. I would like to do more of these, but my teacher only lets me go through the bit she marks.

11.00 We watched a television programme about a farm, where they have lots of cows to produce milk for us. We all have milk every day, but now I know what happens before it comes with the milk-man. I would like to be a farmer, but only in the summer, because I would not like to get up in the dark.

11.30   We had singing, and 'pretending to be things'. My teacher uses the tape recorder and we choose to be animals and things. My friends and I wanted to be fighter jets, but we were not allowed to.

12.00   This is the time for the dinner hour. I had school dinners, but I do not like everything, especially liver. Maybe I will bring a packed lunch next term, because Mummy has been told that hot dinners are changing to something called 'buffet', and prepacked dinners. If I bring my own I can have all the things I like, and it will be like having a picnic every day. My friends and I can swap things too. Mummy says we can plan my picnics at the weekend for the whole week, and put them in the freezer with the days marked on them. I like this idea, because I can choose like a grown-up. We played in the playground until afternoon school.

1.30   We had painting and model making first of all. I did two paintings and made a model. If I only do one painting it might have to go on the wall, so I do another, so that I can take one home. My model was of a tank with big guns on the front. Roger made one too, then we had a battle and smashed them up. My teacher said we were silly, but it was fun, and everyone laughed. Well everyone except Mrs Williams.

2.30   We had another playtime, and I fell over and hurt my knee. I had to go inside and have some cream put on it, but I do not like plasters, because they hurt when you pull them off. Mummy says you should let the air get to things, and they will get better quickly. I quite like seeing the blood, especially when the girls make a fuss.

2.45   We had a really good story today about wizards and magic. It was quite frightening, that is why we all liked it, and my teacher lets the story last for a few days, so that we can look forward to the next bit. In case we do not remember every-thing, Mrs Williams tells us quickly what happened yester-day, or asks some questions about it, and those who can remember can answer them. If we want to, we can draw a picture whilst we listen, because it is difficult for some of us to sit still at the end of the day. Mrs Williams says 'You must have ants in your pants'. That is a bit rude for a teacher I think.

3.15 I walked home by myself, although I saw my brother with his friends, we did not walk together. Sometimes Mummy meets me, not because I'm too small to go home myself, but because she needs to go shopping, or feels like a walk. On such days I may have some money to spend in any shop I like. I might buy sweets or an ice-cream, or save it towards a toy that I particularly want. I save for my holidays by putting some money in a money-box, and sometimes a 50 pence piece appears like magic. I think it is Daddy who puts it there, but he says it must be goblins or something. Only girls believe in that sort of thing.
When I got home I had a drink and played on my bicycle until teatime.

5.15 I watched Dr. Who, which is always exciting. I watch Blue Peter too, and cartoons, when Daddy joins me, if he gets home in time. Sometimes we all have a meal together, and sometimes my brother and I have our tea, and my parents have a dinner later on. It is nice when we eat together, otherwise this only happens at weekends, and we do a lot of our talking and listening to each other at the table. For a treat we have a TV supper, but only if there is something special, or my parents are going out, or having friends in for the evening. In this way we all have a treat, even though we have to be especially good. I like speaking to visitors in a grown-up way, which is allowed before I go up to bed. Sometimes I get out of bed and listen to the grown-ups downstairs. I thought it would be exciting, but it sounds very boring, and nobody takes any notice, so I go back to bed and play with my soldiers until it is time to go to sleep.
I must have gone to sleep at some time because the next thing I remember, it was morning again.

SEVEN YEARS OLD: AN OVERVIEW

Seven-year-olds reflect a growing awareness of their environments, and of their own identities within. Compare the art work of a 5-year-old, with a similar child of 7, and the details which are realistically represented have developed considerably. Relationships between objects, accurate colouring, space relationship, a base line concept upon which all else depends, and time representation may all be seen through art work. At 3 years old 1 % of children will draw a base line, by 6 years, more than 50 %, and by the age of 8 years, 96 %. Allowing for the normal distribution range of intelligence, this points towards a 100 % figure for children within that normal range, or above it. Those below would understandably reflect a delay in this emerging concept, as in many others.

Another interesting method of representing space or a journey, is for children to draw the view they may see, from their own points of reference in their own pictures. This results in the total picture containing portion or portions, either upside down, or sideways to the viewers. Sometimes sides of buildings are 'removed', so that the view illustrates what is going on inside. Hills and slopes may still have trees, houses or people arranged at right angles. Proportion and perspective usually reflect the children's subjective view of their own world. Things will be shown as seen personally. A plate of food will stand on its side to show what is seen by the diners themselves. Important items within their world will be of special size or colour. Characteristically, the completed work of art will illustrate a mixture of all the concepts mentioned. Such pieces of art are fascinating to collect and use for source material or joint discussions.

Seven-year-olds will be interested in behaving and dressing like an adult, not only in imaginative play, but as part of their natural social development. They will have accepted that there are different role adaptions according to situations. For example, people often adopt a 'telephone voice', and will sit or stand in a particular way according to where they happen to be. It would be unusual to see a middle-aged couple sitting cross-legged in a restaurant, unless it was an Eastern establishment! The 7-year-olds will elaborately cross their legs, and smooth their clothes in one mood. In another, they will sit, legs splayed, on the floor, They are beginning to appreciate that codes of behaviour vary according to the social mores within their own society.

The 7-year-olds' familiar wail of 'It isn't fair', or 'You don't love me', are a reflection of doubts experienced as self image continues to be established. It may be related to the common doubt of parentage felt by nearly all young people at some stage. 'Am I adopted?' is a question most parents have been required to answer at some stage, and it is often posed quite suddenly.

Best friends are an important facet of everyday life at school, especially for girls. They change fairly regularly, but there seems to be a very real need to have one, most of the time. Maybe this is another illustration of the 7-year-olds' apparent need for security and protection. To explore and experiment with a best friend reduces the risk of criticism or failure, 'A trouble shared is a trouble halved.' Joining groups such as cubscouts or brownies satisfies the urge of many 7-year-olds to 'belong', and be identified by uniform, badges, and 'secret' signs, or specific knowledge. Collecting of badges is accompanied by collecting of all sorts of other items as widely ranging as can possibly be imagined. Alongside the traditional stamps and souvenirs, collecting such things as flowers, comics, dolls, music boxes, books, records, and many more, can be the start of a life-long, and even lucrative hobby and interest.

The acquisition of knowledge by young children which is linked to their hobby, can be more advanced and demanding than either their teachers or parents would imagine possible. If this drive to learn, associated with individual interest can be harnessed to other basic skills, it is obvious that with an acceleration of such skills development is possible.

Within a normal class-size group of 7-year-olds there is an amazing range of physical and intellectual profiles. This obviously presents a challenge to the teacher, who strives to provide a programme aimed towards the optimum development of each child, in each of the familiar areas of growth. Another point worth remembering is that children vary within these facets. For example, a seemingly immature 7-year-old may be of superior intellect. A well-socialized child, who presents a mature image due to being an only child, could well be a slow learner. As the human child proceeds through the period known as childhood, still relatively protected compared to other species, typical profiles demonstrate the variations rather than a norm. Characteristics become applicable to a whole chronological span, and any specific stages become logically related within a sequential pattern, rather than to an accepted or identifiable age.

PETER IS EIGHT. PETER'S ACCOUNT OF HIMSELF

'Usually I am so busy, that I do not have time to do boring things like tidying toys or cleaning my teeth, or eating breakfast quickly enough, to get ready for school properly. This causes problems, but then I can always catch up if I do it all very, very fast. But then it appears you cannot do things well, if you hurry, so my mother and father say. It seems I cannot win, so I just let them nag at me for a while, and life goes on quite happily.

I do not really have time to go in for moods or arguing like girls seem to, so I might thump about, or kick something. Of course my favourite thing to kick is a football, and I would like to be a professional when I grow up. Mum and Dad do not seem very keen on this idea, but their's always sound pretty boring including words like prospects, security and qualifications. I think it would be great to earn a lot of money doing what I like best, like Kevin Keegan. I belong to a school team, and another at the weekends, and I like training with the other boys. Dad helps to train the Saturday team, he's a good goalkeeper, but I prefer running about all the time. Sometimes we have to take my younger brother with us, but this is a nuisance, because I do not get enough time to talk to Dad, like men together.

One of the things that worries me sometimes is the fact that in other countries, boys the same age as I am, are living in places where there is fighting, and children's parents are being killed. I hope this never happens here. Although I like playing wars with my friends, it's only a game, it does not mean we would enjoy it being real. When we play games, we like to swear or use words we are not allowed to use at home. We have heard some on television, so we know soldiers speak like that. It sounds tough and grown-up. There are also funny rhymes we are not supposed to say, but we do when Mum and Dad and the teachers cannot hear. Some of them are about girls.

I was going to do model making for my hobby at school, but I only wanted to make tanks, and they were not good enough. I do not think the glue was right, because I know I made the model properly. I know because I read the instructions. It is important that I keep very fit for my football, so I do not mind going to bed, although I used to when I was 7. I am luckier than my best friend Jamie because he broke his arm during an important game. At first he was quite proud of his plaster, and everyone sympathized, but very soon it was boring and his arm kept itching underneath. Then he had to use a knitting needle to scratch himself. I have not broken anything yet, but two or three of my friends have.

Both my Mum and Dad have said, that they are pleased that I am so grown-up now. We enjoy doing things together, like visiting places on holiday, as long as they do not dawdle. I like to have a look at everything, and then do something else. They talk with me about things more, rather than leaving me out, and even listen to my ideas. I like that. In fact I can even tell them something they do not know, like when they could not find a shop on holiday, and I remembered where it was. I am good at remembering, like knowing the names of cars, and the way to places. I'm better than Mum at doing that sort of thing, I expect that's why Dads usually take such responsibilities, and I'm getting ready to be one.

One of the best things about being 8 is that I can be grown-up, or a little boy, according to how I feel.'

SUMMARY

The whole stage of development covered in this section reflects an era of attractive, interesting growth. Normally, any problems are

NB Although convenient to scratch with knitting needles, it should be noted that they are sharp, especially the metal type, and should be handled carefully and kept out of reach of young children.

overshadowed by the endearing characteristics of childhood. It becomes clear that children are not small replicas of their parents, but independent beings, capable and enthusiastic in creative and original thoughts and actions.

It is also clear each individual may only develop according to a recipe of environmental and genetic criteria. Although most babies will present very similar behaviour patterns during the first few weeks, allowing for basic personality variations, these variations widen as special aptitudes emerge. One cannot and must not expect parallel behaviour at any parallel chronological age. This is of course presupposing, that the range of normality has been allowed for. It would be ridiculous, for instance to assume that 'all normal 3-year-olds should not necessarily be independently mobile'. They should.

Between the ages of 3 and 8, young human beings have normally achieved a degree of personal independence. Indeed during the early 1800s they would probably have been contributing to the support of the family, by going out to work. Socially and economically this is no longer required of them, but they still have the potential to do so. This is worth considering when one looks carefully at the typical 8-year-old of today.

Chapter 6
Development Digressing from Normal Patterns

Although it has been stated quite emphatically that there is a wide variation in the rate of all aspects of development, there are many children who will fall outside this range of variation. These particular children may be termed as those with 'special needs'. It is the responsibility of those who care for, and about, the young, through careful and intelligent observation, to record the signs which indicate that there may be more deviation from the norm than is acceptable. This applies to all aspects of development.

Diagnosis is obviously the responsibility of highly qualified and experienced professionals. These may be of the medical, psychological, or educational world, and often the experts from various fields will make joint decisions. The most important aspect, however, is the early detection of any warning signals. Those equipped with a first class knowledge of 'normal' human development will be best able to notice warning signals at the earliest moment. This is one of the reasons why nursery nurses are obliged to practise the skills of observation during their planned learning period. It is only with constant observation exercises, and familiarity with normal healthy children, that the skill of detection of small deviations becomes efficient. Sometimes it is difficult to state precisely why there should be concern about a child. The well-experienced person may only be able in 'nonspecific' terms to express an uneasiness, resulting from very small deviations from normal behaviour. In isolation, each example will probably be accepted, but a combination is just not acceptable.

For example, a child learning to communicate will present amusing combinations of language such as 'I'm getting learning of going in the lines, aren't I'. (Kathryn 5 years—after trying to write on lined paper.) If she constantly confused the structure in such a way

89

there may be a problem. If a 2-year-old boy bumped into something now and again it would be normal behaviour, as body coordination became refined. If he bumped into things all the time, then some investigations should be carried out. There is a fine line between a clumsy child and a mildly palsied child, the latter sometimes being labelled the former. Once again, a person with an experienced eye would recommend that the child could possibly have more of a problem, than that of being clumsy.

Some of the more familiar examples of children with special needs will be looked at in this section.

HEARING LOSS

Sounds are measured in decibels (dB), the following is an approximate indication of their relationship to familiar sounds: 20-30 dB, a whisper; about 60 dB, a speaking voice at a little over 1 m (about 3-4 feet); 100 + dB, a close pneumatic drill. Somewhere between 120 and 140 dB is the threshold of pain. Hearing loss when diagnosed, can range from mild to moderate, severe, and finally profound deafness. It is 'one of the most desperate of human calamities' (Samuel Johnson). When there is little or no response to any sound, the loss is of 95 dB or even more. It may be that the problem is not one of strength of sound, but of pitch, when an individual may not hear either high or low pitched sounds. People with this problem often hear a voice better on the telephone than in normal conversation. This is because when one speaks on the telephone there is a tendency to present a level tone and to speak more clearly.

High tone loss causes difficulty in hearing consonants, low tone loss causes similar problems with vowels. Imagine language without one of these properties, or read a passage without sounding them. This is what language may sound like to these individuals. Obviously children who have pitch loss react to the amateur tests for deafness carried out by parents. All babies of 4 months should be tested properly by the experts at the local clinic.

Sound is transferred by vibrations which arrive at the outer ear. These pass along the canal to the drum, the division between the outer and middle ear. This organ is connected to three tiny bones in the middle ear, which is about the size of a Malteser. Vibrating, these bones pass the sound to the cochlea in the inner ear. This organ contains the auditory nerve endings, the main vessel of which carries the message of sounds to the brain.

Three or more children per 1,000 have a hearing problem severe enough to be termed a handicap. About one of these will be due to unknown causes which is about a third of the total. About a quarter are genetically determined, similarly about a quarter are due to illness. The remainder can be ascribed to causes either before or at birth. German measles of the mother early in pregnancy can cause serious defects, amongst them deafness. Severe jaundice can result in deafness after birth. Often children with hearing loss are multiply handicapped.

After testing, a hearing aid is often recommended. There are many different types and they must be fitted professionally, and maintained in a similar way. One of the drawbacks of a hearing aid is that it magnifies all sounds, and the child has to learn to select what he or she requires, a very complex skill. Even if the young child is fortunate enough to be diagnosed early, most have to wait and so lose the first few months of valuable early language experience. Obviously this cannot be replaced, and an effort must be made to compensate, by offering more than usual in the way of sounds and language.

Most children, even with hearing loss, will have some residual hearing, and many can be educated in normal schools, others may even have access to special units attached to normal schools. Those who require very specialized help for most of the time will be educated in 'special schools'.

Deaf children tend to have more emotional problems than those who hear properly. Understandably the frustration of not being able to communicate, is deeply felt. More tantrums have been observed in preschool children with hearing loss. More effort is required to make oneself understood with a deaf child, and it is easy to cut short the conversation and make do without achieving successful communication. This will only intensify the frustration already experienced, and prevent the child from developing his or her own individual language potential.

Nursery nurses may find themselves in the position of being able to give time and attention to children with hearing loss. They should remember to follow carefully the advice offered by the specialists, and to observe and record in detail expected progress, or lack of it.

VISUAL LOSS

As with hearing loss there is a wide range of visual loss. Mild loss can be corrected easily, by wearing individually prescribed glasses. These are much more readily accepted than hearing aids, and can contain very powerful lenses, before drawing any attention from other children.

Visual loss is easier for the amateur to suspect, and even to confirm. Obviously no precise diagnosis can be made, this is the job of the specialist, but it is clear if a baby does not respond to a smile, or reaches out without locating visually, that expert help should be sought. All such school age children are divided into those 'partially sighted' and those 'blind'. The decision is usually made solely on the criterion of whether the child will be able to learn to read from print, or whether even with magnification, reading is impossible and the learning of Braille is required.

Causes of visual loss are similar to those of hearing loss. German measles is again a familiar culprit. Genetic inheritance and accident at birth contribute also. In the third world, blindness in some areas is much higher because of the organisms in untreated water.

Parents who learn that their child is visually impaired, will obviously need help and support. Some local authorities have assessment teams. Failing this, the Royal National Institute for the Blind have a team of advisers who travel all over the country. The team, unfortunately, is small, but useful information is available from the RNIB.

It is helpful to put the parents in touch with another family who are experiencing or, even better, have successfully experienced coping with a child who is visually impaired. They will be in a position to advise the 'new' parents, who will be emotionally very vulnerable. They will be able to recommend courses of action, avoiding the long process of trial and error which can be frustrating and demoralizing.

As mentioned, the visually impaired baby does not respond to smiling. It has been observed that the vital bonding between mother and child proves much more difficult under these circumstances and this should be appreciated.

Blind children follow the same developmental pattern as sighted children although the rate is usually slower. For example, sighted babies walk, because they are aware it is a useful skill to acquire. Blind babies need to be given the idea. The nursery nurse will sometimes have a child who is visually impaired. By following the advice and instructions of the specialists much can be done to encourage the areas of development which would normally proceed at a natural pace without visual problems. Blind children will be cared for in a special environment and the skills required in this situation will be acquired whilst working there.

EDUCATIONALLY SUBNORMAL CHILDREN

As a result of the 1944 Education Act distinctions were made between children who as a whole group did not present an intelligence quotient (IQ) within what is accepted as the normal range. The most common intelligence tests indicate an average score as 100; 68 % of any normal population will achieve scores fairly evenly spaced between 85 and 115. This is accepted as 'normal'. The 1944 Act grouped educationally subnormal children, usually those achieving 70 or less on IQ scales:

a those of limited ability.
b those retarded by other conditions such as illness, or regular absences.
c those ineducable or severely subnormal (SSN).

The first group scored 20 less than the score expected for their age; the second, more than 20; the third would be probably unassessable on the normal accepted intelligence tests. The scores mentioned are intended as a guide only, and it should be remembered that each child will be individually examined and other aspects of behaviour and performance will combine to provide the material for any diagnosis, and for any decision-making. Again as a fairly rough guide an individual's IQ may be calculated as follows:

$$\frac{\text{mental age}}{\text{chronological age}} \times 100$$

Therefore, a 10-year-old child whose mental age is assessed at 15 will score an IQ well above average

$$\frac{15}{10} \times 100 = 150$$

Genius level starts at about 140. When a child has a serious problem, it is easier to diagnose, come to terms with, and commence appropriate treatment. If the problem is marginal the parents will naturally delay any decision-making, in the hope that their child is a late developer, or a slow learner. Many famous and very learned men have recorded poor achievement early in life. Sir Winston Churchill's early development gave no indication that he would develop into one of the greatest men in history.

Educationally severely subnormal children ESN(S) are classified in Britain as those scoring IQs of 20-50. There is distinct delay in all areas of development.

Educationally subnormal children ESN(M) have IQs of 50-75 and may not even be diagnosed, but will be slower to develop language and motor skills. It is obvious once again that skilled observation is the key to diagnosis and, in turn, the key to early professional help. The value of the practice of detailed, recorded observations must never be underestimated. They are vital to the future of those young children, whose problems must be diagnosed as early as possible. Only a very thorough knowledge of normal growth and development is sufficient preparation for this practice.

It is not clear, nor universally accepted, that there are specific reasons for mental retardation in, by far the larger proportion of these children. Some are obviously brain damaged, as a direct result of accident or disease or even environment. For many the causes are an obscure combination of hereditary and environmental factors. They do however present some common characteristics. Amongst these the following may be observed:

1 Long delays in encountering, and successfully passing through, the familiar developmental stages.
2 Difficulty in handling abstract concepts.
3 Very short spells of concentration.
4 Problems in making sense of messages received through sight,

sound and touch, although physiologically the organs function efficiently.

5 Inconsistent memory ability.

6 Understanding may well not relate directly to the ability to express thought.

In extreme cases of this nature a symbolic language may be learned. Makaton and Bliss are comprehensive sign languages used for communication when there may be problems such as spasticity or mental retardation. Joey who was severely spastic and lived at St Lawrence's Hospital in Caterham, Surrey, was a prime example of such a problem. His ability to speak was severely restricted and it was not until another patient succeeded in responding appropriately to the sounds he made, that it was realised how mentally able Joey was. He has written a book reflecting the tragedy of frustration suffered by those who simply cannot make others understand.

Children of subnormal intelligence do present a very wide range of behaviour problems, some bordering on normal 'naughtiness', others tending towards the bizarre. There is a constant dichotomy between those who advocate integration of handicapped children into normal schools, and those who insist that special facilities should be separate. It must be remembered that the child with behaviour problems will demand much of the teacher's attention, thus drawing it away from the rest of the group, who may suffer, continuously. One way in which some authorities offer a solution is for children who require special care, to be catered for in a unit attached to a normal school. These children may then integrate when appropriate, but will not interfere with the normal learning programme of the rest of the school.

Very often children who are educationally subnormal need the sort of care which would be appropriate for children younger than themselves. The greater the problem, the greater the age difference for such an approach. For example, a child with marginal difficulty could be happy and make progress in a remedial class, where the curriculum is simply taken at a slower pace with much more reinforcement at each stage. A child with severe difficulties, whose development is some years behind the norm, will need the care appropriate to a much younger child in all areas. Naturally the older the children become the greater the social problem. As they begin to grow into adolescence they will present as physically mature people very often with the attendant language and behaviour grossly mismatching their physical stature. Although they are not in any way dangerous, their family understandably may well begin to isolate them more and more in social terms. This can affect the whole family, brothers and sisters sometimes suffering considerably as they themselves are growing up. Such families need much support, and in the fields of overstretched resources, such as those of the mentally handicapped, this support is frequently inadequate.

In 1974 the government set up a special committee to inquire into the education of handicapped children and young people. This was chaired by Mrs Mary Warnock and a report was published in May 1978. One important recommendation was that the existing categorization of handicapped children should be replaced by a new concept of special educational needs. This lays an obligation upon the education authority to provide an appropriate special education based upon the needs identified for each child. A particular child is never labelled with a specific disability. Also the report embodies a positive statement describing the type of special education required at a specified time.

The term 'educationally subnormal' was to be discontinued in favour of 'children with learning difficulties' and that the term 'handicapped children' was to be replaced by 'children with disabilities or significant difficulties'.

Recommendations made by Warnock were introduced by the government through legislation in 1981.

CEREBRAL PALSY

The range of variation found in cerebral palsied children is vast. From one extreme there is often reference to chronic clumsiness, at the other, the child is unable to achieve control of any muscle groups at all. Such children are often handicapped in other ways, many being aurally and/or visually impaired. A lower than average IQ may also be found.

A cerebral palsied child is afflicted by a nervous system where messages breakdown between the brain and the muscle. The latter simply fails to receive the message, and therefore cannot carry out the instructions. It is rather like having permanent pins and needles, although this familiar sensation is not actually felt by the cerebral palsied child. About three quarters of these children are also spastic. This condition renders muscles rigid and stiffness of the limbs cause disorganized movement. The term 'spastic' is frequently used in a very generalized way which is incorrect.

About 1 in 600 live births presents a cerebral palsied child. The cause is rarely hereditary and is usually attributed to prenatal environmental factors, or injury at birth, or later in life. There is no cure for a palsied child, but treatment in the form of therapy helps the child towards his or her individual potential.

Those who care for such children can play a vital part by following carefully the directions of the physiotherapist, speech therapist and occupational therapist. The time spent in sessions with these professionals is of limited value, unless the work is carried on with the child as a part of everyday life. Once again an intelligent awareness of human development is necessary to be of maximum help to the child.

It is relevant to point out again, that many severely affected children may 'hide' an intelligence above the normal accepted average.

EPILEPSY

Attitudes towards the epileptic have probably caused suffering equal to the problem itself. In biblical times those affected were accused of being 'possessed of the devil'; in mediaeval times probably of the similar related crime of 'witchery'. Women may have paid with their lives for suffering from epilepsy. Even today there is a common fear of being faced with the problem of someone having 'a fit'. It is disturbing for the onlooker, but needs to be understood much more widely, to lose some of the associated fears.

An epileptic fit has been described as a 'thunderstorm' in the brain, a disorganized electrical patterning. This is reflected by the familiar body reaction of stiffening, spasms, loss of consciousness and muscle control. The latter often causes incontinence during fits.

There may also be some breathing difficulty. This type of behaviour is called grand mal or major sickness. A less dramatic form known as petit mal or minor sickness, is characterized by what are known as 'absences'. When affected in this way, children may appear only to lose concentration for a brief period, they may cease to focus visually, and be accused in the classroom of 'dreaming' or 'switching off'. In this way many may not be accurately diagnosed.

In Britain there are about 60,000 children liable to have fits, most of these can be educated in normal schools, their conditions being controlled adequately by the regular administration of suitable drugs. About 600 attend special schools, one of the largest being in Lingfield, in Surrey.

Factors causing some individuals to be liable to fits, and not others, are not very clear. Sometimes brain injury follows accident or illness, but in the majority of cases the cause is obscure. The tendency, however, once it does exist, can be exacerbated by increased stress, and it has been known for children to induce fits, and even to enjoy the experience. First aid treatment for a fit is to ensure that the patient can breathe, remove any objects which may cause injury, place the patient in the recovery position when appropriate, and in many cases allow the patient to sleep comfortably afterwards.

The everyday care of children who have epilepsy should, in principle, emphasize normality, whilst being prepared for the incidence of fits. Such children should never be alone for long periods, nor should they be exposed to sharp changes of light as these can induce fits. Examples offered are: flickering television sets, bright sunshine through trees when travelling in a train or car, disco lights. It has been known for young children to simulate such conditions using their hands in front of the sun. Such activity would be observed by the skilled person, and some action taken.

There is no reason why children with epilepsy should not swim. What should always happen is that they do so in the presence of someone who knows about their problem, and they must appreciate this. In special schools, such children wear a cap of a particular colour so that teachers may easily keep these children under observation. Many people with epilepsy lead normal lives, they may drive cars, and hold down the job of their choice. Many more will probably do so, when there is a wider understanding of the illness and a greater appreciation of the enormous range of its nature.

DIABETES MELLITUS

Diabetes usually conjures up the image of daily injections and portions of food being carefully weighed at each mealtime. Diabetes is a condition in which the body is unable to process efficiently starch and sugar. It is inherited.

Sugar and starch are normally converted into energy, which is distributed to the various body organs in the form of glucose through the blood stream. This conversion is controlled by a hormone called insulin, produced in the pancreas. This hormone travels through the blood stream to points in the body where glucose will enter the tissue releasing energy. Excess glucose is stored as fat although a little may pass through to the kidneys, where it will normally be extracted causing the urine to be glucose free.

If the system does not operate efficiently, insulin is not produced so the glucose is not converted, and this presents the kidneys with more than they can cope with. In this situation glucose will be found in the urine. As glucose carries water more urine may be passed. In turn the individual will drink more presenting a recognizable symptom of the disease. Obviously the energy which the glucose ought to be providing is missing, so the sufferer feels the need to eat more, another familiar symptom.

Diabetes may be developed in childhood, adolescence or middle age. It is not present at birth, and only about 1 child in 12,000 is a sufferer. Although there is no cure, diabetes can be effectively controlled, by offering insulin to compensate for the body's failure to produce it. This is usually injected for children, although tablet form may be offered later in life.

This medication, however, is not the whole answer, as the body will not be able to adjust the intake of insulin as it would if naturally produced. Simple testing of the urine is necessary three to four times daily. Diet and exercise need to be regulated as obviously exercise will use energy quickly and the adjustment problem presents itself. At these times warning signals such as sweating, loss of concentration, difficulty in speaking or reading, or tearfulness, will indicate an urgent need for glucose. This may be administered by offering sugar, chocolate or sweets, usually with speedy satisfactory results. Once this first aid treatment has been completed a meal should follow within a short period of time. For obvious reasons a child with diabetes should never be kept waiting for a meal. If the condition does not receive attention, the patient may become comatose in which case medical attention should be sought as an emergency. Some children have unfortunately used this method of attention-seeking often when experiencing the developmental problems associated with adolescence.

The reverse problem develops if the system is presented with too much sugar, when the patient is unusually thirsty or hungry, feels tired, breathes deeply, and has a sweetish breath. This condition develops slowly, and to alleviate it, insulin is administered. Diabetics should always either wear a bracelet or necklace containing medical details, or carry a card offering similar information. As with other conditions children should be able to attend a normal school happily. It is necessary for those caring for such children, in whatever situation, to be made fully aware of the needs of these young people. The more they know the more confident they will be, and more able to handle any of the related problems which may occur. It is often the ill-prepared adult, and not the child, who causes a situation to become disproportionately stressful.

CLEFT PALATE/HARE LIP

During prenatal development the roof of the mouth of the upper palate normally joins up, together with the upper lip. Sometimes this process fails to be completed and the cavity of the mouth is not properly separated from the nasal cavities, and is known as a cleft palate. This obviously presents sucking and feeding difficulties. A hare lip is an ugly deformity and most upsetting for the mother. The condition is caused by the upper lip failing to close at the centre during prenatal development. Fortunately surgery always results in a beautiful baby, the scars being almost invisible. This operation is usually performed at about 3 months.

A cleft palate is repaired once each side of the palate has reached a uniform size, usually at a few months of age. Up to this stage a plate is fitted and renewed as necessary. This is designed in such a way as to encourage even growth, as the growth at birth is usually uneven. If even, a plate will not be required, although it does help the baby to feed more easily. A cleft palate affects the development of clear speech, so children affected will normally require therapy.

There is some indication that a cleft lip and palate may be caused by hereditary factors. Whatever the cause the deformity develops during the first 3 months of pregnancy. Some babies seem to breast-feed successfully, others can cope with a bottle, and both can be tried with some optimism. Special spoons, however, are also available, either attached to a bottle or separate, but feeding by this method can take a long time. Babies should be held in a more upright position than normally recommended, as this helps to prevent food entering the nasal cavity. This is most unpleasant for the baby, and he or she may approach feeding with some apprehension. The main thing for parents to appreciate is that, however shocked and resentful they may be when they see their baby, the baby is unaware of any problem. In fact he or she will never, due to the miracle of surgery, have to see his or her deformity, or be subjected to any expression of horror.

Surgeon, dentist, audiologist and therapist will be part of the team who will help and guide parents and child. Once again it should also be emphasized, that each child will present a unique set of problems, that each develops at a different rate, and therefore treatment recommended will most likely vary from child to child.

THE AUTISTIC CHILD

It is impossible to offer a clear characteristic which would enable simple diagnosis of an autistic child. Rather it would be a collection or set of criteria which found together would present a picture of autism.

In simple terms, these children are not able to 'make sense' of their world. They may react inappropriately to sensory stimuli, move about in an incongruous way, and reject attempts made to socialize them. Autistic children also tend to resist change and a regular routine seems to be preferred almost to the point of obsession.

One familiar activity is that of repetitive short movements, like flapping hands, opening and shutting things, or banging.

Currently accepted criteria in the UK for the definition of autism are:

1 An onset before the age of 5,
2 Autistic type failure to develop relationships with people,
3 Abnormal language development,
4 Ritualistic and stereotyped behaviour.

The cause of autism is not yet reliably established. Autistic children need skilled help in all forms of learning which they seem unable to acquire through imitation. The observation of activity seems to have no link with the children themselves. It would be useful for the reader interested in this particular affliction to read *Dibs : In Search of Self* by Virginia Axline and *For the Love of Ann* by James Copeland. The future for autistic children is bleak. Many find themselves in special hospitals and most are unable to lead an independent life when they reach maturity.

A sad, but interesting point is that there appears to be no record of an autistic child having children. There is a view that autism may be caused by parental 'coldness' or inability to create a satisfactory emotional environment for their child. Although some cases seem to emanate from an emotional trauma, there is no evidence to support that any parental shortcomings can be responsible for the development of autism.

Parents will naturally have feelings of guilt, however unjustified, when they realize that their child is not developing normally. When no blame is due, this cannot be emphasized strongly enough.

ASTHMA

The child who is subject to attacks of asthma is probably suffering from an allergy, the body is overreacting to something in the environment. This something may have been touched, eaten, or inhaled. Eczema and hay fever are also illustrations of allergic reaction.

A tendency to allergies often runs in families and is therefore hereditary in many cases. In spite of this pattern, the symptoms may not present themselves in a similar form. For example, a child with eczema may well have a parent who is asthmatic. The process of allergy may well alter through the life cycle, many problems reduce as the child grows older. Likewise if the child is unfortunate enough to display two allergic problems simultaneously, one will often improve whilst the other becomes more serious.

A child with an attack of asthma can present a very frightening picture. In simple terms, the bronchial tubes become narrowed, and there is considerable difficulty in expelling the stale air from the lungs. This results in the familiar noisy gasping and panting. A relatively high number of children in the UK are asthma sufferers, the estimate is as high as 1 in 20. This of course will cover a wide range, from those children experiencing an occasional attack, to those whose attacks may even last several days.

The substances which cause an allergic reaction are numerous, among them are pollen, house dust, fur, feathers, or certain foods. When exposed to any of these the child who is particularly vulnerable to one or maybe a combination, may suffer from hay fever, asthma, or allergic conjunctivitis (puffiness, irritation and watering of the eyes). Stress can also precipitate an attack of asthma, although psychological causes are not to be considered solely responsible. Due to the acceptance of the effects of stress, however, children who are sufferers should be kept as free as possible from situations which would raise such factors.

It may be necessary to subject children to a long programme of tests in order to isolate the cause of an allegic reaction. These are not usually carried out under the age of 4 years. If tests reveal a clear cause, by the skin reacting to a substance, then a course of injections containing the substance isolated, can desensitize the child. The reaction will then be considerably reduced or eliminated, for a period of time, after which another course of treatment may be recommended. If an item of food is found to be the culprit it can usually be withdrawn from the diet. Eggs are sometimes found to be a problem. Another method of treatment is to reduce the effects caused by allergens by using drugs, such as antihistamines and cortisone. The bronchial tubes can also be dilated and relaxed by using inhalers.

These should always be used under the direction of a doctor, and the adult who cares for the asthmatic child should seek medical advice on the use of inhalers. These aids should not be overused.

Bronchial asthma

When a child is suffering from bronchial asthma the symptoms relate closely to wheezy bronchitis. In each there is difficulty in breathing out efficiently, thus expelling all the stale air from the lungs. Although the treatment in both cases is similar (physiotherapy, drugs or medicines) it is necessary to discover which cause is giving rise to the symptoms. Wheezy bronchitis often disappears by the time the child reaches school age. Asthma, however, may continue and may have hereditary connections. The latter will often present itself without warning, whilst the bronchitis often commences with a seemingly normal cold.

As with many other conditions, *remember*, above all, to calm and reassure the child and if he or she is able to understand, explain what is happening both whilst he or she is suffering an attack, and during treatment.

SPINA BIFIDA AND HYDROCEPHALUS

The most common serious congenital abnormality of *spina bifida* presents itself in a variety of forms. Simply described, there is always some deformity of the spinal column in which the bones, in some way or another, fail to fuse completely, and the spinal cord may protrude. If this happens the cord protrudes into a sac, and the child may suffer paralysis and a deformity of the lower limbs, numbness, incontinence, kidney infection, and will probably be intellectually handicapped.

On the other hand the child least affected will lead a perfectly normal life. Sadly for the child seriously affected, there is no cure.

Hydrocephalus is often associated with spina bifida and the child suffers from a build up of fluid in the brain. In 1958 for the first time, a shunt, containing a valve, was inserted to drain the surplus fluid, and this dramatically improved the quality of life for affected children. A surgeon and an engineer developed the instrument calling it the Spitz-Holten.

When caring for a child fitted with a shunt, the danger signals are:

1 Fever, vomiting, bad temper, loss of appetite, may indicate that there is some infection,

2 Headaches, vomiting, sleepiness, possibly a fit, may indicate a blocked valve,

3 A swelling behind the ear or along the tube may indicate that the shunt has become disconnected.

Observation of any of these, or a combination, must lead to an immediate request for medical advice. Further information may be obtained from the Association for Spina Bifida and Hydrocephalus, Tavistock House North, Tavistock Square, London, WC1H 9HJ.

COELIAC DISEASE

The fairly rare condition of coeliac disease produces the symptom of large pale motions which are offensive. This is due to an inability to digest fat, due to the presence of gluten which is ingested through wheat flour and grain. When a gluten-free diet is established the child develops normally. Other symptoms of this condition may be wasting of limbs and buttocks, hair is thin and in poor condition, and a susceptibility to infections. The condition usually presents itself between 1 and 4 years of age. There is no cure for coeliac disease, but the dietary treatment is effective.

CYSTIC FIBROSIS

The disease, cystic fibrosis, is inherited through a gene carried by the parent's chromosones, although they themselves may not be sufferers. The problem is due to the mucous glands oversecreting, and causing the ducts to become blocked. The digestion of fat and protein becomes impossible, and the child appears to need much more food than normal. The stools are loose, greasy-looking and offensive, and the child is probably underweight and pot-bellied. The child may also be wheezy because the mucous produced in the chest tends to gather there. The untreated child could become a respiratory cripple, but antibiotics can be effective. Research is being carried out into treatment through diet, and some encouraging results have been observed, often feeding children with predigested foods in the form of beef serum, together with added nutrients. Physical activity and breathing exercises are also recommended.

RICKETS

In the condition of rickets, the bones fail to develop properly and actually soften and bend. This is due to an inadequate supply of vitamin D, which is converted through natural sunlight. Some foods such as margarine have added vitamin D and others such as fish oil contain this element.

It is not wise to offer too much vitamin D to a young child, and once a good mixed diet is established there should be sufficient taken in to withdraw supplements. When vitamins are administered, however, it should be noted that children with dark skins need more as they naturally filter out much of the sun's rays, which would allow conversion into vitamin D.

DOWN'S SYNDROME

It has been explained the ways in which an extra chromosome appears in the genetic patterning of individuals affected by Down's Syndrome (see p. 9).

These individuals are physically distinctive. The head is smaller than normal and appears flat at the back, and the eyes slant. The ears sometimes lack all the familiar curves and creases and the hands are short, especially the thumbs. There may be a large gap between the 'big' toe and the next. The condition may be diagnosed immediately after birth due to these clear physical characteristics.

All those affected suffer some degree of mental handicap, and most are prone to chest infections, partly due to the flattened bridge of the nose causing fewer infections to be efficiently rejected. These babies lack muscle tone, the limps being floppy and unable to respond. In most cases of Down's Syndrome, the mother and father are genetically normal, however in some cases there will be some abnormality carried by the parents, who should then receive genetic counselling in order to determine future risks.

Chromosome tests on the amniotic fluid are likely to indicate whether or not there is an abnormal chromosomal patterning, but it should be pointed out that the results of such tests are not 100 % accurate. Normal readings have resulted in a Down's Syndrome baby being born, although this is rare. These children are very affectionate and on the whole do not present serious behavioural problems. They often live at home and are educated in special schools or units. When they reach maturity many are employed in sheltered workshops and are involved in a social life. Unfortunately they tend to be found in institutions later in life, due to many being unable to achieve total independence.

FAMILY REACTION

It is vital having looked at some of the more familiar types of handicap, to consider the most important people to the child, the family. Obviously there is a vast difference between giving birth to a handicapped child and experiencing the trauma of accident or illness severely affecting a healthy child.

A common reaction to either is that of a failure to understand, a refusal to comprehend. A numbness sets in, information is mentally diverted whilst the body and soul prepare themselves to cope with the shock. This happens to individuals in other traumatic situations such as bereavement. When realization begins to dawn, the next instinctive move is to search for reason, for alternatives, explanations, causes, treatments. This period allows for activity, mentally and physically, restoring a sense of purpose. Things do not seem so bad if one can actually *do* something about it. This is reflected when parents of missing children or other relatives insist on searching, even when it is advisable for those emotionally involved to stay at home and wait, and allow the police to be active.

The next emotion is of anger and blame. This may be specific and directed, or general and undirected. When this period brings no result, there is only despair left, and during this experience the child and family are in desperate need of all the support available, from voluntary, statutory and personal sources.

Hopefully, as a result of such support the situation will be accepted to some degree, and some planning will take place, enabling all those involved to view the future in a more positive and optimistic way. Naturally as wide as the range of handicap or disablement is, the range of personalities taking part in the situation and their individuality will determine how they react and cope. In this way the whole quality of life of the affected child will be dependent upon those making decisions.

The more informed parents are, the better equipped they will be to make those decisions, both for the short-term and long-term benefit of the child and of the family. There should also be constant awareness of all needs: social, emotional, intellectual and moral. Caring for the handicapped child is a long demanding labour of love.

Chapter 7
Special Needs/Special Problems

There is no doubt that some children seem to have difficulty in coming to terms with their environment. They appear unable to synchronize happily whether on a physical, social, emotional, intellectual or moral plane. In modern society it is necessary to harmonize with other members to coexist happily. This does not mean to say that conflict has no place but that such an encounter should either lead to solutions or improvements. Conflict can be therapeutic. Anger properly expressed can achieve positive outcomes. There are many reasons why individual children or groups cannot come to terms with their specific environment in a satisfactory way. Some of these will be looked at in more detail in this section.

It is essential, however, to emphasize most firmly that these children usually present few, if any, problems at all. They may have special needs which may be partially or wholly met but most will adapt to their environment quite happily. Therefore, never assume that, because a child comes from a one-parent family, speaks English as a second language, is left-handed, or adopted, such criteria give rise to problem behaviour or can be used as an excuse for it. Such children are mostly well-adjusted and happy but they will, at some stage, have presented special needs.

Special categories of needs do not provide the necessary prerequisite for special categories of problems. They are though, sometimes related.

MINORITY GROUPS

Under the classification of minority groups will be found immigrants, travellers and service families.

Immigrants

Immigrant children will be considered as a single case, although it is obvious that second or third generation children will not present the language problems encountered by newcomers to the country.

Language is not the only area demanding attention, even though it is usually the most overt. As a result, it is the area which receives the most resources and the most care. What is often not appreciated is the difficulty children may well encounter in living within two cultures. They are having to make efforts to adapt at school, whilst returning to their natural environment and language at home. Eating habits, dress, religion, cultural family lore and language may well constitute to form an entire microsystem within a home, or area of a town or city. In areas like Brixton in South London, the immigrant community can no longer be truly classed as a minority group.

In school or nursery, special language stimulation is helpful, even for some West Indian children, whose dialect may be difficult to interpret. The efforts of the adults serve a useful purpose, but the most productive time will probably be spent in the company of the other children, during flexible unstructured activities.

Some groups have distinctive modes of dress and diet; girls may not be permitted to show their legs; boys to cut their hair, and later bare their heads. Pork and subsidiary products are 'unclean' to Moslems and may not be eaten.

Travellers

Travellers, if they come to school at all, do have special needs. They come from a cultural group not universally accepted by the rest of society. They take their 'holidays' at unconventional times, live in unconventional dwellings, speak differently, guard their culture almost fiercely, and come and go.

Some schools make provision for these children to remain as a large 'family' group, with a teacher who has built up a special re-lationship with the Romany community. Many of the parents are keen that their children should become literate and numerate in the accepted sense, but they need to trust the education staff in order to entrust them with their children. The teacher will, ideally, make regular 'home' visits, in order that a good relationship is developed.

As a result of their parents' way of life, children who move around at regular or irregular intervals are rarely able to benefit from an educational experience in the same way as those who are settled. Methods will vary from school to school, curriculum content and a readiness to accept children for short periods will also vary. Add to this the fragmentation of any possible programme, and it must be appreciated why many such children voluntarily cease to appear in any formal learning establishment, after primary level. Secondary education is rarely, if ever, seen as relevant to their particular way of life.

Service families

Another group who are obliged to move around during their years of formal education, are children of service parents, and civilians employed abroad, or in different locations in this country. It is true to say that continuation is assured through provisions made here and abroad. Continuation, however, does not necessarily indicate sequential progression. Such is our system that schools are most unlikely to be following similar programmes at similar times. In some European countries all children in the same year will be encountering the same lesson at the same time. This obviously has some arguable disadvantages due to its inflexibility, but it does remove some of the problems which could be encountered by children who move around.

SUMMARY

Any child who, for one reason or another, moves through many educational establishments will require special attention, both academically and also, and most importantly, in social and emotional areas, in order to readjust as happily as possible. Children cannot begin to learn effectively until they are emotionally and socially stable. Consequently those who are unstable in these areas of development are unlikely to achieve their potential. If a child is in a situation where his or her needs are not being adequately met, potential is not realized and he or she may come temporarily into one of the categories and thus present special needs.

One of the most difficult aspects involved in meeting needs is that the child is part of a family group, and that group has much more influence than any other institution. To solve the problem for a few hours each day, is like sticking plaster over a wound which needs stitching first. Even if it is impossible to work with the family, it should be appreciated that such an aim must be recognized.

ONLY CHILDREN

Most children without brothers or sisters are so through force of circumstance rather than design. Parents normally anticipate a family of at least two children, the pattern tending towards an average family size of somewhere between two and three.

Unless a conscious effort is made to plan time for only children to spend with others, of a similar age and younger or older too, there is often characteristic behaviour requiring modification, in order for them to socialize effectively at school. For instance, sharing and taking turns is a new experience, and one reasonably resented. This behaviour may never have been learned. Listening while other children express a point of view, even tolerating a less elaborate language code, makes demands on an only child who has been given time to speak and has, at the same time, developed a language code more closely linked to that of the adult, than his or her peers. Children with English as their second language tend to have unusual constructive patterns and words woven into their English. It is easy for other children to laugh, making these children reluctant to use the language which they have a great need to develop, in order to benefit from the education programme offered.

Only children may be labelled precocious and lacking in respect for adults. This is usually due to a failure to appreciate that these children have probably been used to discussing issues with adults, much more than children who have siblings. They also often participate in the social life of their parents at an early age. One extreme example, well-publicized some years ago, was Ryan O'Neal's daughter Tatum. She was smoking and attending late night parties with her father at a very early age. Photographs illustrated the sophisticated way in which she was dressed for such occasions.

It is said that parents make all their mistakes with their first children. Only children, it would follow, are products of parental experimentation and mistakes. Although this rarely causes any severe problems, fortunately, it should be remembered when caring for only children, that they do have special needs and require sensitive understanding. Integrating happily into a peer group makes considerable demands on their adaptability.

CHILDREN FROM LARGE FAMILIES

Children from large families usually know how to share and take turns as part of their everyday life. There may, however, be a fierce competitiveness to rise within a 'pecking order'. This 'order' depends on the background culture of the individual family. In some, the male will be afforded priority whatever the age; in others the reverse will be found and ladies will come first. It can be useful to be the eldest or the youngest, again depending upon the inherited cultural attitudes. Even allowing for the development of equality for both sexes, within the family, those from cultures other than our own especially, still hold discriminatory attitudes.

Boys are frequently allowed more social freedom, even in areas of sexuality. Education is still deemed more important for boys in many mixed families. If there is sufficient finance to send some to a private school, the boys may well be afforded such a privilege, on the basis that the girls will 'only get married'. Children from large families, for obvious reasons, often have less in material form than only children, or children with one sibling. Unless there is real poverty, this does not seem to be a handicap.

Traditionally and naturally, most good parents ensure that their children are well-fed, clothed, sheltered and loved. This security causes them to view the material goods that wealthier friends may have, in a balanced way. It is the parents' role to educate their children not to envy others; not an easy task, but necessary for future contentment as 'Men will never be equal!'

Parents of large families may be partners in a second or even third marriage. This often causes stress and strain both for adults and children as a result of the complex sets of relationships experienced. The children are always the unwilling victims of parental stress, and even if no physical or emotional abuse is intended, there must be some suffering. Emotional security is threatened when the adults in a child's life show signs of instability, and this may be reflected through antisocial behaviour. Children simply cannot express the fact that they are distressed, because their mothers did not speak to their fathers for 2 days, or because their mothers' attitude towards them has altered due to the pressure of money problems. Their world has become insecure, and they may attack it, or withdraw from it. In any case their relationship with the world becomes distorted, and thus their behaviour and attitudes towards it.

What seems to be so often misunderstood is that young children do not enjoy behaving in a disturbed way; it does not make them happy. Therefore, shouting, punishing or restraining, only serves the immediate needs of the adult to achieve some control. It may be necessary to do this for the sake of the other children, but do follow up as soon as possible with positive support, and specially directed attention—ideally on a one-to-one basis. Do not leave a child alone with his or her unhappiness.

Children from large families, however secure, will benefit from individual attention which is difficult for them to achieve at home.

TWINS/TRIPLETS/QUADRUPLETS

The benefits and drawbacks to being born a twin, triplet or quadruplet are relative, becoming more emphasized as the multiple increases. Obviously one of the drawbacks is that there is always another at precisely the same age presenting the same needs, often at the same time. The mother will at times have to cope alone and, consequently, is bound to become more tired, and sometimes more stressed than a mother with one baby, or even a baby and toddler. It follows that each child of a multiple birth is likely to receive less individual attention.

Language development may also be affected and twins especially have been known to 'invent' a special code through which they communicate effectively, but which their parents are unable to understand. More often there may be a little delay, due to the fact that the twins have less need than a single child to communicate with adults.

Twins who are identical and are dressed in similar fashion have been known to record later in life that they suffered some loss of identity. Common reference to 'the twins' in itself tends to reduce their individuality but is usually the term used. Comparisons are always made, wisely or otherwise, between brothers and sisters. Twins are unreasonably expected to perform in a similar way, either academically or physically. There is no reason for fraternal twins to follow such a pattern and it can cause feelings of inferiority to develop when one twin is markedly less able in some specific area. Identical twins, however, often develop similar specific skills, as reflected in the world of sport. The Rowe twins were champion table tennis players and the Bedser twins top class cricketers. Twins do not necessarily develop matching skills and talents.

LEFT-HANDED CHILDREN

Historically, association with the left has questionable connotations. In heraldry, for instance, anything on the left is called 'sinister', which itself means evil-looking, wicked, unlucky or threatening.

Until the 1930s or 1940s most children were encouraged, persuaded, some even forced, to use their right hand, even when there was obvious preference for the left. Some behaviour problems have been ascribed to such practice, i.e. stammering and nail-biting.

It takes a left-hander to appreciate fully the problems encountered, especially in early life when children probably do not realize why they cannot perform tasks with the same skill and ease as their right-handed friends. Free painting, however, is without such restrictions (Fig. 7.1). Much, of course, depends on how fussy the parent is in areas such as table manners. The accepted way to hold a knife and fork, the former in the right hand, does not usually come naturally to the left-hander. When using a single implement, the left hand will not only be preferred but will obviously be more efficient. Most people will not even notice the soup spoon being passed over to the left.

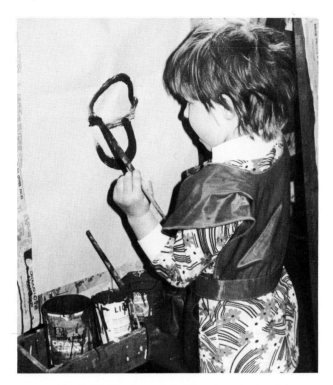

Fig. 7.1 The left-handed child (above) is holding the paint brush in a more mature fashion than her right-handed friend (facing page).

Another problem when learning to write is that left-handers would be happier working from right to left. They have to overcome such a desire and arrange themselves physically so that they can actually see what they are doing. Observation will confirm that adaptation has taken place and either the paper is turned almost at 45° or even more, or the arm encircles the paper and the hand 'drops' down over the top of the page. Another method is to write from underneath the line being worked. As a result of acquired habits, some children produce pages of writing which seem to change character every few lines. This causes the finished work to look untidy to say the least. Sometimes it even looks as though more than one person has done the work. Observe the child actually engaged on the task in order to understand the problems encountered.

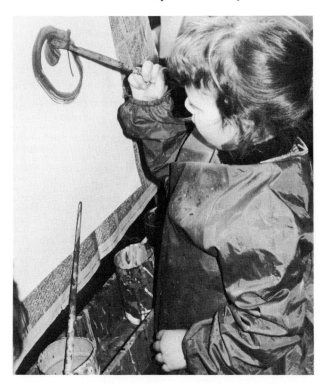

Other areas of difficulty are tying shoelaces into bows, sewing, knitting, using some tools, e.g. potato peelers, shooting, playing some games. Some of these skills are relatively simple to learn from someone who uses the same hand, others require adapted tools. There is no escape from the fact that life is geared towards the right-handed. Therefore a little more understanding of the left-handed learners, especially at an early age, is necessary for them to transfer the skills required into their individual methods of execution. Diagrammatic instructions are often very difficult indeed to follow in reverse.

Left-handers, it must be noted, are very useful sportsmen and women, often having similarly useful ambidextrous tendencies, and have been known to be skilled at writing backwards (mirror writing).

It will be clear well before school age whether a child is going to be left- or right-handed. This preference is often indicated during the second year of life by kicking a ball using one foot much more than the other. Do not confuse kicking with the earlier activity of simply 'walking into the ball' when the foot used will be equally left or right.

Apart from the few social and adaptive problems faced by left-handers, they develop happily, achieve similar goals to their right-handed contempories, and certainly should never be persuaded to 'change hands'. Their brains will follow a specific developmental pattern which is designed to match the left-handedness indicated.

CHILDREN FROM BROKEN HOMES

It is an unfortunate, yet a common misconception, that children from 'broken homes' will present more problems of a serious nature, and there is a tendency for it to be used as an excuse by children and adults alike. No-one would deny that the events leading towards termination of a relationship can be traumatic. No-one would deny that the period immediately following such an event can be dominated by problems outside the experience of all parties concerned, thus causing severe stress.

However devastating it may appear, most families do manage to adapt to the new situation and to lead positive and even happier lives. It would be dangerous to generalize about such serious experiences and, of course, for many the healing process is a long and difficult one. For some it is never complete and one partner will suffer in a similar way to the bereaved, who are unable to come successfully to the end of their mourning period. For the children of such parents there is obviously a great need for emotional security, just as for those whose parents are unable to communicate successfully about their children's future, care and control, custody and access.

Another group at risk emotionally are those whose parents remarry and have another young family. It is not difficult to imagine how the children of the first marriage must feel under such circumstances, especially if they spend some time with each parent.

There are many combinations of outcome to the 'broken marriage'. It is rarely an experience without pain and some bitterness. What must be considered first, and the law seems to agree, is the safety of the children. Security should be seen in the areas of physical, social, emotional and moral security. All can easily be threatened and each is interdependent to ensure positive and balanced development. The victims of broken marriages are the children and parents who remain alone after the break. In most cases this situation emerges: very few partners both re-establish themselves immediately. In nearly every case also the remaining unit will be unable to maintain their accustomed style of living, in spite of everything the legal profession may say. This is particularly so when there is an economic period during which wives and mothers are working to provide an adequate standard of living, rather than the luxuries hitherto traditionally aimed for.

Children from broken homes need support, understanding and comfort. They do not need to be so sympathetically treated that unacceptable behaviour is tolerated or excused. There is no reason for them to abuse individuals, property or society any more than other children. Expecting and accepting such behaviour certainly does any such child a disservice and will almost surely cause them to encounter more problems, rather than less, as they grow up. They beg consistency, not flexibility to the point of absence of direction, which is what many of them are served.

FOSTERED CHILDREN

There are two categories of fostered children, those in short-term and those in long-term fostering situations. The former usually come into care for a brief period as a result of some serious problem at home, e.g. mother may be in hospital, she may be suffering from stress, the child may be at risk physically.

A child is usually placed at short notice and, therefore, adequate preparation is impossible. The foster mother must be very carefully chosen and will need to be extremely sensitive to the possible reactions of a child suddenly removed from home. In many cases there is insufficient time to build up a proper relationship; the resentment frequently displayed by the child has to be anticipated and accepted. Successful foster parents are special people who seek no immediate reward, and open their homes and family life to unknown and possibly very difficult visitors. For it must be appreciated that the work is a team effort and successful fostering is only achieved in such a way, the whole family being united in their effort to offer a child, even for a brief period, the security they themselves enjoy.

Long-term fostering often means a child living for a period of some years with foster parents. These children become a very real part of the family, and links with their natural parents may fade as time goes by. There is usually a definite reason for such children to remain fostered and not be adopted. The most common is, that parents are unwilling to make the final decision to relinquish all rights of control over their own children. Of course, once a child is legally adopted, the adoptive parents are obliged to accept all responsibilities, including financial ones. It could, therefore, be that if a child remains legally fostered, financial security is maintained more adequately than if he or she was adopted. There may be instances where there is no possibility of a child being removed by a parent, and will remain fostered to enable a family to carry out their fostering satisfactorily and at the same time remaining financially stable.

There may be many suitable families who could offer long-term or permanent care in their homes who nevertheless feel that they are not in a position to meet the extra financial burden of adoption. A large number will view fostering as rather a precarious arrangement but enquiries would confirm the number of children who, although not available for adoption, are most unlikely to be able to return to their natural families.

Fostered children do not necessarily present specific problems or require special treatment. According to each individual case they do deserve an understanding watchfulness on the part of those caring for them. There will be times when coming to terms with the world and the people in it asks more of the children than they can produce at the appropriate times. For one reason or another they have not received their quota of loving and security, so a little extra emphasis in either or both, is thoroughly justified.

CHILDREN WITH CHILDMINDERS

Childminders have become, to a large extent, the hidden mainstay of the day care service for young children. Those registered with the local authority, a legal requirement, only represent a fraction of those women actually caring for other people's children on a daily basis. The number of immigrant families concentrated in some city areas, reflect a cultural habit of minding children for parents who must go out to work. They do not appreciate, with some justification, why local authority officials should monitor their activities.

There are, however, situations in which there is serious exploitation of the shortage of statutory facilities. Many children may be cared for under cramped and dangerous conditions. There may be insufficient heat, unsuitable nourishment, and few play opportunities. It is necessary to operate some official register aiming to ensure that certain standards are maintained. Research indicates that the system fails to highlight the inadequate standards which exist. Official procedures and form-filling tend to reduce enthusiasm for many exercises, and there is a very large number of first class childminders providing a vital service who have remained unregistered.

Children who spend their days with 'good' minders (it is not intended to qualify here the criteria desired) probably have the best of both worlds if their mothers cannot care for them every day. They have the stability of home and parent or parents, they have good substitute care, together with the opportunity to socialize with other adults and children. Such children may develop well in all areas of independence.

It is necessary for mothers/fathers to build up a good relationship with their childminder. In this way any contrasts between care can be minimized. It is one of the advantages of such a personal service that method and practice can be of an individual nature, rather than the institutionalized pattern found in larger establishments. Another advantage is that minder and parent can become friends in a real sense, and the children will observe and benefit from this. Also that the minder is much more likely to remain a constant figure for a longer period of time, than in most institutions. Added to this, if the child needs to be looked after outside the conventional working hours, a private childminder is in a position to cater for this. She or he may even be able to continue care when the child is mildly unwell, a problem not usually accepted by statutory establishments.

The biggest disadvantage is obviously the varying standards of private childminders. Most mothers can judge whether or not they would be happy to have their children in a specific environment, with a particular person or persons.

It is worth pointing out that there are cases of maltreatment and unprofessional conduct brought to the courts every year. These usually relate to the parental home or official institutions where young children ought to be safe. Prosecution of a childminder is extremely rare.

REJECTED CHILDREN

Rejections can probably be handled successfully from friends, acquaintances, even siblings. Parental rejection is another matter and total distortion of normal development can result. First of all it must be understood that those who reject their own children are themselves in need of help. Their own development has become distorted, as normal, healthy development should lead to good parenting; it is the natural outcome of stable, balanced experiences.

Many reasons are offered to explain rejection, i.e.:

a Sex of the child not accepted,
b Unwanted pregnancy,
c Close resemblance to a divorced partner or disliked member of family,
d Child who is 'different'—details often not explained,
e No logically expressed reason.

The latter is probably the most common of all, even if the parent can admit to the rejection which, in itself, means some progress on the road to acceptance.

Human beings need to hold a good image of self; this affects totally their behaviour and attitudes. Rejected children see themselves of little worth and, consequently have a very poor self-image. In order to improve this image they will automatically experiment with a variety of behaviour styles. They will assess through the reaction or attention of the adults in their life which pattern elicits the most attention. Obviously the situation becomes one of a spiralling nature. The more antisocial or bizarre the behaviour, the more rewarding the response will be. Even when the response is accompanied by physical abuse, the child still seems to feel the exercise is worthwhile. Some children become withdrawn and cease to communicate at all. Either type of reaction of extremes will require specialized help and treatment. Such treatment will probably be carried out through regular sessions at a Child Guidance Clinic or Special Clinic attached to a hospital.

To have maximum effect these children will need support during most of the week, month or year, depending on the length of the therapeutic programme. Those responsible should follow the advice of the professionals as closely as is practicable. Obviously if the parents are involved at an early stage, so much the better. They may be ready at some other stage to participate and the door should be constantly open at all times for such a partnership to become established. The adolescent boy who states that his parents never really wanted him, may well be interpreting what was actually the case. Sadly he is unlikely to be stable and well-adjusted, is probably working through problems alone, and is unlikely to know how to be a good parent himself. So, once again the cycle of deprivation is illustrated.

CHILDREN OF WORKING MOTHERS

There are more mothers than ever before going out to work, either part-time or full-time. For many it is no longer to pay for luxuries such as holidays but to maintain a reasonable standard of living for their family in times of high inflation. It may also be, to substitute for the lost income of the traditional provider, the male of the family unit, who is unemployed for one reason or another. In a few instances traditional roles are reversed and the male will adopt the role of caring for the children at home during the first few years of their lives. Children of such parents, although their mothers work, do have the benefit of constant care at home.

Another category receiving constant care at home is those looked after by nannies, mother's helps and au pairs. Such arrangements are usually successful, but it should always be appreciated that foreign au pairs will be unable to encourage and foster language development in the same way as a mother. This is due mainly to the difference in language use, but also due to a very basic difference in emotional ties. Au pairs rarely spend more than a year or two with a family and one of their chief objectives is to improve their own language fluency in a second tongue.

There is bound to be some difference between the home of a working and nonworking mother, especially for the school child. A working mother will not always be at home to welcome or meet the child from school; she will probably have to spend part of the evening cleaning or washing as well as cooking; she will be tired and, consequently, unable to give the children the time and attention they need. Such children may be required to help with domestic chores at an early age. This is not harmful as long as the children are able to keep up with school work, sleep sufficiently, and socialize within their peer group. On the contrary, the acceptance of some responsibility within the family group is a good foundation for future life.

Children of working mothers will sometimes arrive at school without essential items, or those required for a special activity. These children should not be criticized or punished automatically, their mothers may simply have forgotten or had insufficient time to make adequate preparations. Similarly there are the children who 'forget' to bring something for the bazaar, 'cannot' have a costume for the concert, 'leave' their packed lunch at home. Their problem is compounded by their natural loyalty, and more often than not, the real reason for their 'carelessness' is an overcommitted parent. It is important to know as much about the children in any care situation as possible. Only then can they be fairly treated at all times.

CHILDREN WITH HANDICAPPED SIBLINGS

Owing to the large range of handicaps and the intimate combinations which together may affect a child, it is impossible to be specific. The thoughts here, therefore, must be of a generalized nature.

It is natural for parents to try to compensate for any handicap their child may suffer. When such children have no brothers or sisters this is an easier programme to follow. All available human and financial resources may be directed towards such compensation.

When there are brothers and sisters, understanding and sympathetic though they may be, there is a danger due to this very altruistic tendency for them to become neglected. This type of neglect results from sacrifices being made by the whole family. The attention of parents, relations and friends is often focussed on the handicapped child, little notice being taken of the able sibling. The able are expected to do well at school, behave better, be less demanding and unselfish. After all they are gifted in relative terms, they are 'normal'. The family may go out together on rare occasions, with or without the disabled child. Babysitters are more difficult to find, and taking the child can be physically and/or socially difficult.

The able sibling may, therefore, lead a very restricted life in social terms. Holidays may be impossible. Even when handicapped children are in weekly residential care, the weekends become totally dominated by arrangements for them to travel home, spend some time there, and travel back.

Although it is nearly always after considerable heart-searching, that young handicapped people are placed in long-term residential care, the result on the rest of the family can be very positive indeed.

ADOPTED CHILDREN

The story of adoption is usually one of success. If a child is adopted by a family of similar colour and culture at a very early age, only the normal range of needs should be demonstrated as the child grows up. This is, of course, accompanied by the normal range of problems, no more, no less.

Special needs may understandably be displayed by those adopted late in life, or by families from another culture or of a different colour. The former will probably have experienced rejection more than once and possibly numerous times. There may have been years of instability and/or abuse, physical or emotional. Their self-images need to be established or restored, together with trust in adults.

There are a few instances of coloured children being adopted by 'white' families. The reverse is almost unknown. Obviously these children realize the difference at an early age, and questions need to be answered as fairly as possible. These children will also experience questioning from other children and adults as they socialize and go to school. It is surprising how tactless adults can be, even those who are supposedly well-educated. The children should be prepared for such events with suitable responses, avoiding the real temptation to challenge the question.

The biggest decision for some adoptive parents is when, or if, to tell the child. Legally an adopted person over the age of 18 is allowed access to information in order to trace his or her natural parents. Many feel the urge to do so, even though they do not intend for a moment to transfer their loyalty. Some adoptive parents find this difficult to accept, but curiosity is a strong drive, not uniquely held by the very young.

A problem sometimes met in adolescence by adoptive parents and the adopted person is that typical behaviour is not accepted. The parents see it as behaviour that 'a child of their own' would not present and place the blame on the natural unknown background. The young person sees this as rejection and blames the parents for adopting in the first place. The ensuing rift can be painful enough to cause separation even of a permanent nature. All parents of adolescents appreciate the 'stranger' emerging from the rather lovely son or daughter who frequented the house only a short time ago. Only experience will produce confidence in the phrase 'All things must pass'.

There is support for parents for the immediate period following adoption. Many would probably welcome more, at later stages of development.

Chapter 8
Child Protection

SAFETY

Adults who care for children, whether their own or other people's, are totally responsible for ensuring that their environment is as safe as possible, and that when this cannot be controlled the child is protected, and then educated to respect danger and behave accordingly. Accidents are the biggest cause of death and injury to young children. The number who suffer as a result of traffic accidents together with those which take place in the home, present unacceptable figures, which can to a large extent, be reduced drastically. This is due to the fact that human error and carelessness are often the main cause. The first step therefore is to inform and educate, the most essential groups being the future parents, and those caring for other people's children.

Home

THE KITCHEN

The kitchen is one of the most potentially dangerous places in the home. The materials which cause burns, scalds, cuts and even drowning are found here.

It is better if young children are not allowed freedom of movement during working time in a kitchen. They may be in a playpen, under observation in a hall or other separated area, or safe in a high chair, playing and watching. If outside they could play within view, or take fresh air, and rest in a large pram. Later, young children can join in by working or playing imitative games.

There are several precautions which will make the kitchen area safer. The cooker should be fitted with a guard, which will prevent containers falling off, and fingers helping them to do so. All handles should be turned inwards, and spoons should not be left standing in pans. Kettles must not be overfilled and left to boil. Water, as it expands, will spurt out of the spout or lid and fall to the floor. Remember too that electric hot plates look black, when they are still dangerously hot to touch.

Electrical appliances should always be disconnected and the flex folded up and put away. The sockets must be of the special safety pattern, with shutters, and if possible should be out of reach; often sockets in all areas are placed near to ground level. Flexes need to be carefully positioned so that no part is left to hang over the side of a work top, shelf or table. Likewise table cloths are best avoided, table place mats are just as attractive and provide less washing if spills occur, which they frequently will. Spills on the floor should be mopped up immediately for the sake both of safety and hygiene. Knives should be kept in a safe secure place, even locked in a drawer. The magnetic holders look attractive but when viewed with all those sharp points facing downwards, the question of total reliability of such appliances must be raised.

Washing machines and tumble dryers or spinners are more often in the kitchen than anywhere else, and do present both fascination and danger to the toddler. Water becomes very hot, depending on the type of wash, and spinners do not stop instantaneously when lids are raised. Toddlers have drowned in machines containing a few centimetres of water, others have been severely scalded after falling in.

If the telephone or door bell rings, take the child out of the kitchen. Another familiar hazard is the low cupboard, often under the sink, where so many families still keep cleaning fluids and other household materials which can kill young children, or at best cause distressing sickness, and necessitate unpleasant treatment. Receptacles used for rubbish are frequently at ground level and easily entered by the toddler or crawler. They often contain glass, opened tins, empty containers with contents still inside, and spoiled food. There is no need to elaborate on the possible consequences of a few minutes alone, with such a collection for a young child.

THE BATHROOM

Once again as in the kitchen the hazards in the bathroom are obviously those of hot water and cleaning preparations with drugs and cosmetic aids added. There may also be a socket for an electric razor.

Although it is common knowledge that electricity and water will cause electrocution of a body partially or wholly immersed, there are still regular incidents of such accidents. Usually an electric fire has been taken into the bathroom, and falls into the water. Better to suffer a cold bathroom however spartan this may appear. It is easy for a small child to slip over in the bath, so a special mat, nappy, or piece of towelling can be placed under his or her bottom to create a fairly efficient anchor. Even so, young babies or toddlers should never be left alone, they may be able to turn the hot tap on, or may slip and go under the water. Although at best they may just have a fright, at worst they may be scalded or drowned. This is not alarmist, such tragedies have been recorded.

It is worth mentioning at this point, that all medicines and tablets must be kept in a secure place, preferably in a locked cabinet. Some of these medications are most attractive, looking like sweets, or fruit drinks, and a very small amount of either can cause serious damage. A mixture may easily be fatal. It is surprising how many responsible and well-informed parents have had children who have managed to eat or drink drugs prescribed for a member of the family, and who had to be rushed to a casualty department as a result. Accidents happen to children of caring, responsible, well-educated parents, and they feel the sense of guilt as much as anyone else, if not more so.

DOORS

Doors made mainly of glass have caused horrific injuries when children or adults have fallen through them severing veins or arteries.

STAIRS

Stairs are another potential danger area, due to the natural instinct of toddlers to climb. They are not sufficiently able to anticipate the results of the action, to know that the higher they climb the longer the drop. A guard gate at the top and bottom of the stairs may ensure the safety of a toddler or creeping baby.

Similarly small children, when observing those swimming in deep water will not appreciate the total situation and have been known to jump in, and to their surprise, disappear. A sense of danger takes time to develop, and this, just as with all aspects of development, occurs at different rates. It must never be presumed that children, because they have reached a certain chronological age, can be made responsible for specific aspects of their own safety.

HEATING APPLIANCES

In the UK it is necessary to provide artificial heating in buildings for a large proportion of the year. Some systems present more safety problems than others. Open fires and paraffin heaters are probably responsible for most accidents by fire, both to persons and property. Cigarettes are also high on the list of causal factors. Many if not most, and probably all, of these tragedies could have been prevented. Some of them result in multiple loss of life, whole families of young children being victims.

A recent case involved a fire in Mid-Glamorgan where a stepfather and 5 of his children died. They were trapped upstairs when a fire broke out in the dining room at the rear of the house. The mother and one child escaped by jumping from a bedroom window.

Open fires, gas fires, electric fires, fan heaters, paraffin heaters and radiators should have the appropriate guard protection. This should carry the British Standard Safety Label, which guarantees a quality of design and workmanship. This label is awarded after rigorous testing. Radiators have been mentioned, because they can become hot enough to burn young skin. Children must never be left alone with open fires or paraffin heaters. When the weather is cold it may seem harmless to pop out for a few minutes, but it is potentially dangerous.

WINDOWS

Windows can be fallen through, so it is a wise precaution to fit vertical safety bars which can be removed as the children grow up. Simple observation will confirm that very few houses do have such fittings. It is fair to say also, that few accidents do occur through children falling from windows, probably because the hazard is so obvious, and therefore natural caution is effective. Balconies with low walls are probably more of a potential danger.

FLOORS

Generally speaking floors should be even, and nonslip. Rugs should not be placed loosely on polished areas. All areas especially close to steps or stairs need adequate lighting, and the control switches placed so that it is unnecessary to walk any distance in the dark, either to turn the light on or off.

Outside

Even whilst babies are still in their pram they may be exposed to various dangers outside. Cats possibly attracted by the smell of milk find it warm and comfortable inside a pram and may well settle on the baby. A very young baby can be suffocated in this way. Fit a cat net, even if there are few cats around, it only requires one, to jump into the pram, to result in possible tragedy.

When babies are sitting up, they will probably enjoy rocking their prams, which is great fun. The serious danger here is that a pram can actually travel an amazing distance in a short time as a result of this rocking. It can end up by falling down a slope or steps, or by causing damage to the car. In the first situation the result needs no further elaboration, in the second it can be frustrating and costly. Make sure that the stationary pram will remain so.

As the child becomes mobile the normal environment will present hazards. Poisonous berries and fungi, milk bottles on the step, insecure gates, broken washing lines, workshops and garages containing harmful fluids and tools, stray dogs, family vehicles and careless neighbours, to name but a few. The adult needs to evaluate these potential hazards from a child's point of view. A view motivated by an insatiable curiosity drive. If in doubt err on the side of caution. It is unlikely that the child will suffer from overprotection, there is ample opportunity in today's world to experience danger and take risks.

ROAD SAFETY

The term *road safety* trips off the tongue rather too easily and some of the presentations to young children are too humourous, or tend to romanticize the process of safety in traffic. In reality there is no large handsome hero to pull the careless child out of danger, no dressed up squirrel to remind children to take care. Let the child be guided, then guide the adult, then display and prove competence.

FIRST AID

In case the worst happens and an accident occurs it is advisable for all adults, but especially those responsible in any way for young children, to be able to administer first aid treatment. The main areas of accident are heat—burns and scalds—fractures, asphyxia, bumps and bruises, poisoning and bleeding.

Heat injury

BURNS

Burns are caused by contact with dry heat and electricity. From 450 to 500 children die in the UK every year from burns and scalds in the home and most of these could have been prevented. Up to 11,000 such incidents require hospital treatment as an inpatient.

Sunburn comes in the dry heat accident category. It can be serious in young babies and small children. It is not commonly appreciated, that even strong sun reflecting off a window onto a baby can cause sunburn, serious enough to require medical treatment.

SCALDS

Scalds are caused by wet heat such as boiling water, steam, corrosive chemicals or any hot liquid. Burns and scalds affect the tissue in the same way and similarly the treatment is the same.

The injury may be first, second, or third degree; all are very painful. All types of burn should be immersed immediately in cold water, or held under slowly running cold water for about 5 minutes. Alternatively a flannel holding cold water, renewed as it warms, can be held over the injury. If there is no blistering, petroleum jelly or paraffin gauze should be gently applied, after patting the area dry. Never rub such wounds. If there is blistering after using the cold water, again pat dry, and cover with sterile dressing or freshly laundered tea towel or handkerchief. Medical advice is then necessary. If a large skin area is affected fluid loss could be serious therefore offer half a cup or so of water every 5 to 10 minutes until help arrives.

The electrical burn may appear minor but can in some cases be more serious, even third degree. Therefore all such burns should be referred to a doctor as should minor burns covering large areas, and a small burn to a very young child or baby. One of the most obvious reactions to any injury is that of shock, and part of all first aid attention is that of treatment for shock, even as a precaution, in case symptoms are delayed.

Shock

Some or all of the following symptoms may be present in shock.
1   Draining of skin colour,
2   Rapid, weak pulse or very slow pulse,
3   Cold, clammy skin, sweating,
4   Distressed respiration, shallow rapid, even gasping,
5   Thirsty, nauseous, even vomiting,
6   The patient will probably be restless, apathetic, and will certainly be afraid and need reassurance.

If any, or all these symptoms present themselves, during calm, constant reassurance lay the child flat, loosen clothing, and cover with a light blanket. Do not attempt to warm the child, this drains the blood away from vital body organs towards the surface, and causes heat loss. The sweating could also cause heat loss, and loss of fluid. If in doubt do not offer drinks as the patient may require an anaesthetic. A child in shock should be treated as an emergency and transferred to hospital immediately.

Fractures and dislocations

A fracture may be suspected if there is pain, immobility, deformity, and swelling. A dislocation occurs as the result of severe twisting of a joint. If it is difficult to decide which has taken place, always treat as a fracture.

If the patient is not bleeding seriously, can breathe comfortably, and is able to communicate, avoid any unnecessary movement, treat for shock and summon medical assistance. Whilst waiting, immobilize any affected limb, by applying bandages or other suitable material above and below the injury point, avoiding pressure on that point. An arm may be tied to the chest, a leg to the other leg. Splints should be applied if the patient has to be moved before a doctor arrives. These should be long enough to extend well above and below the injury point and need to be padded to avoid direct contact with any injured tissue. One type of fracture which should not be moved under any circumstances unless by a qualified first aider, and then only if danger is imminent, is any related to spine, neck or skull. Simply treat for shock, and reassure whilst waiting for qualified help.

Asphyxia, breathing difficulty

There may be difficulty in breathing if suffering from a cold or being in a stuffy or smoky atmosphere. Asphyxia occurs when insufficient air is inhaled into the lungs for one reason or another. There is lack of oxygen through the bloodstream to the brain and carbon dioxide builds up in the bloodstream. If this condition is not successfully treated unconsciousness and eventually death will take place. Four minutes can be sufficient time for the brain to be starved of oxygen for this to occur.

In cases of asphyxiation there will not be time to summon help, and speed of action is vital. First of all after clearing obstructions, apply mouth-to-mouth or mouth-to-nose resuscitation after locating pulse and/or heart beat, or even whilst doing this. Every second counts. The priority is to push air into the lungs and this effort must start at once. For instance if a child has lost consciousness in water, do not try to get him or her out, unless he or she is obviously breathing. Start mouth-to-mouth resuscitation in the water, supporting his or her head.

The ideal position for the patient is flat on the back ensuring as far as possible a clear airway. Pull the jaw upwards and forwards. Standing, kneeling or lying beside the child, take a deep breath (with an older child, pinch the nostrils too), seal lips over the mouth and blow until the chest rises. If the child is very small seal the lips around the mouth and nose. When the mouth cannot be opened, hold it closed and breathe through the nostrils only. Move away from the child by a few inches and listen for expelled air. In a small child administering twenty breaths a minute should be aimed for. For a teenager however, ten to fifteen is about average. In each case the first four or five breaths should be administered at a much quicker rate. If after ten to twelve breaths there is no change in the child's condition and the first aider is qualified, the pulse should be looked for. If there is not a pulse, cardiac massage must be started. The unqualified should continue artificial respiration. It cannot be over-emphasized that all those caring for children especially, should become qualified first aiders. Ideally all adults should attend such courses.

If breathing is inhibited by a foreign body and the child is choking, probably on a piece of food, turn him or her upside down, and slap sharply a couple of times between the shoulder blades. If the child is too big for this hold him or her over a knee, chair or bed, so that the head is lower than the body, and slap sharply in a similar way.

A child may also stop breathing as a result of holding his or her breath, having a fit, inhaling vomit, being trapped in smoke, being gassed, playing with plastic bags. All such incidents demand prompt action as described.

Bumps and bruises

All normal healthy children as they develop mobility and refine motor skills, will sustain some bumps and bruising. The danger is, that those injuries which demand special attention may pass by unnoticed. Such injuries as bumps to the head, resulting in drowsiness or unconsciousness and showing swelling should be referred to the doctor. A tendency to bruise more than usual could be checked with the doctor, also any bruise type marks, which seem to appear without cause.

Poisoning

Accidental poisoning can almost always be prevented. Certainly within the home, there is no excuse for a child succeeding in consuming tablets, medicines, or other harmful substances. Food poisoning may, however, be purely accidental, or at worst neglectful. If it is suspected that a child has consumed a harmful substance there are steps to be taken immediately. Remove any unswallowed items from the mouth, and if possible identify the substance. Then call the doctor or, if he or she is unavailable, take the child to hospital, or call an ambulance. Even during the waiting time it is possible to take first aid action. Remember time is valuable, it can mean life to the child.

Never try to induce vomiting if the child is unconscious, or if a corrosive volatile liquid has been drunk. In the former situation place the child in the coma position. If it is advisable to induce vomiting try tickling the back of the throat with a finger. This is easier to recommend than to carry out. The physical method of inducing vomiting should always be used. A demulcent is a soothing drink offered after, or in place of an antidote. The best are milk, egg and milk, a tablespoon of olive oil in milk or a thin lemon barley drink.

The emetic of water with salt or mustard formerly recommended could complicate medical treatment for poisoning.

After urgent life saving treatment has been administered, in any situation always treat for shock, and always reassure. Keep some of the poisonous substance to show the doctor.

Bleeding

Many people are frightened by the sight of blood, or so they say. Clearly they themselves are not in danger, unless the blood is their own. What should give rise to fear is the knowledge of what may happen to the victim of injury if bleeding is not arrested, and controlled. It would be useful, and at times life-saving, if all adults were skilled in first aid techniques of dealing with bleeding, calmly and efficiently.

If the blood from a wound is spurting and of a bright red colour, it is coming from a damaged artery. If it is dark and seeps more slowly, a vein is involved. In either case apply direct pressure. A clean piece of fabric should cover the wound, but the bare fingers will do if none is available. Raise any affected limb above the head level of the patient, when possible. The bleeding should decrease under pressure, if it seeps through any dressing apply another on top. Do not remove the first one.

Some older manuals recommend the application of tourniquets, but these can be dangerous when applied by the unskilled, therefore the direct pressure method should be used until medical assistance is available.

For small cuts clean the wound in warm soapy water, dry gently, and cover with a clean dressing if necessary. Plasters tend to prevent rapid healing, and this is best encouraged when the wound is exposed to the air. If protection is absolutely necessary during the day, plasters could be removed during the night.

If a deep wound has been caused by a nail or similar object in the garden or playground, it may be a good idea to check whether the child has had a recent tetanus injection. A booster may be recommended, although tetanus is now rare in this country due to routine immunization. If a person had never been given tetanus protection and subsequently suffers an injury which necessitates such protection, this may only be offered by an injection of horse serum, which has a high risk of reaction. If there is any bleeding from nose, mouth or ears, after a fall, medical advice must be sought immediately.

Nosebleeds usually look worse than is really the case. Sit the child upright, leaning the child slightly forward to avoid blood running down the back of the throat. Pinch the nostrils gently if the bleeding continues for 4-5 minutes. Seek medical advice if bleeding continues for more than 20 minutes.

Bites and stings

Stings from bees or wasps are unpleasant but unless the victim is allergic to such accidents, the treatment is simple. The bee may leave the 'sting' behind, and this may be removed by a scraping movement with a fingernail or the edge of a nail file. Direct grasping of the sting will cause more poison to be released. A solution of bicarbonate of soda should be dabbed onto the wound. A wasp sting should be treated by dabbing with vinegar, thus neutralizing the alkaline nature of the venom. If a child is stung inside the mouth it is wise to seek medical advice, as any swelling in this area can prove dangerous.

ANIMAL BITES

A bite from a dog in this country does not carry the danger of rabies. There may, however, be a case for a tetanus booster. It is wise to let a doctor see any such injury.

SNAKE BITES

The only snake in Britain which carries poisonous venom is the adder. They have a zigzag pattern along their backs. If such a bite is suspected, do not suck the wound, just reassure, and seek immediate medical advice. The child should be carried and not allowed to walk, as this may encourage the poison to spread more rapidly through the system.

IMMUNIZATION

Young parents today sometimes see diseases such as diptheria, smallpox and poliomyelitis as historical concepts. Thanks to a comprehensive programme of immunization this attitude is understandable. It would be irresponsible to allow the feeling of security to jeopardize such an efficient method of prevention. Prevention is not only better than cure, but in some cases is the only alternative. The recovery of a child from diptheria or smallpox is by no means guaranteed, even in these times of advanced medical techniques.

There are two types of immunity, active and passive. Active immunity is acquired through the administration of a weakened form of the virus. This allows the body to manufacture antibodies, which then act as a natural defence for a particular disease, without the individual having to suffer an actual attack first. This protection may last for a period of one year, as with influenza immunization, to a lifetime, as in the case of diptheria. Passive immunity is acquired through the administration of blood serum taken from a person or animal, who has already manufactured the particular antibodies required. Unfortunately the protection in this case is short-lived and the body of the recipient may react adversely, particularly if the serum has been taken from an animal.

During fetal development the baby will benefit from any immunity possessed by the mother, this passing through the placenta in the bloodstream. This protection will last for the first few weeks of life. During this time the ability to make antibodies is developing and will probably be efficient at about 6 months. This is why the first vaccination or immunization is now postponed until after this time, whereas it used to take place much earlier.

The only antibody which will not pass to the fetus is that of whooping cough, due to the fact that it is too large to pass through the placenta. There are three methods of administering the antibodies which are held in fluid: first by syrup, to small babies, or drops on a lump of sugar, as in poliomyelitis vaccine; second, by placing on the skin with small pressure points applied through needles, without piercing the surface of the skin at all (this is the method used in the case of smallpox vaccination); third, by a conventional injection method, used for the remaining infections. Table 8.1 illustrates the pattern of immunization generally recommended for children in Great Britain. There will always be some exceptions, and the doctor will make the final decision in respect of an individual child.

Table 8.1 A recommended protection schedule.

Age	Vaccine	Method	Comments
6 months	Diptheria Tetanus Whooping Cough Polio	Combined injection Orally	Known as the triple. The whooping cough vaccine may be omitted.
6 weeks after above	Polio (second dose)	Orally	
4-6 months after above	Polio (third dose)	Orally	
During second or third year	Measles	Injection	Two doses at intervals of 3 weeks.
On admission to school	Diptheria Tetanus	Injection	Booster dose.
11-14 years (Girls)	Rubella (German measles)	Injection	To reduce danger to unborn children
10-13 years	BCG (Tuberculosis)	Injection	If not already immune. At least a month should elapse between BCG and Rubella injections.
15-19 years, or on leaving school	Tetanus Polio	Injection Orally	

Smallpox vaccine is no longer offered as a matter of routine in this country but may be recommended if travelling to countries requiring such protection. Whooping cough is a distressing and dangerous disease especially in young babies. There is no immunity passed on by the mother, so any protection acquired is through immunization. As there is some evidence of brain damage occuring after this particular vaccination, although very rare, it has become the accepted practice, to isolate whooping cough vaccine from the diptheria and tetanus. This allows parents to decide, whether or not their child should receive such protection, after being made aware of any research findings published. The family doctor will advise accordingly.

CHILDHOOD AILMENTS

Most children during their first few years of life, will survive the familiar illnesses such as common colds, measles, german measles, mumps and chicken pox, which are all of the infectious variety.

They may also 'catch' head lice at some stage, some skin infection, and react adversely after eating food which contains some harmful bacteria. It is useful to be able to recognize and know how to nurse children with such ailments, as they are always cared for at home, unless complications arise. Common colds are just that, and unfortunately most individuals accept the usual couple each year, or even more. Some seem to be more susceptible than others, and a few fortunate people go for years without suffering from common cold symptoms. The familar signs are sore throat, runny nose, watery eyes, headache, loss of appetite, rise in temperature and a general feeling of malaise. There is no cure and the remedies offered by chemists are normally of a suppressing nature, drying up nasal secretions, and reducing head pain. Warmth, extra fluids and fresh air, together with light nourishing diet will aid recovery. It is vital to observe any further indication of complications, such as upper respiratory tract infections involving the throat or chest. The ear may also become painful, middle ear infections often causing severe discomfort. When such complications do arise, the doctor may prescribe a course of antibiotics. This course must always be completed even if the child seems better after a couple of days. The reason for this is, that any bacteria surviving will develop an increased resistance to the antibiotic, which will therefore be less effective if needed again. The complete course will effectively kill all such bacteria. Finally, do not underestimate the effects of influenza not only physically but emotionally. This virus can cause depression and certainly seems to weaken the whole body system. The limbs and the head ache and the sufferer may well feel very ill. Recovery will commence if there are no complications after 3-4 days, but will probably take longer than a cold. Treatment by antibiotics for secondary infections may be recommended.

Infectious diseases

MEASLES

The first symptoms of measles are closely related to those of the common cold. Sore throat, watery eyes, rise in temperature, fractiousness and probably refusal of food. The incubation period is from 10-15 days and it is likely that first contact with measles will result in a contraction of the illness due to its particularly highly infectious nature. It is spread by droplet infection.

Even before any rash appears, small white spots inside the mouth, called Koplik's spots will permit confirmation of measles. The rash itself may appear on about the third to fifth day, or sometimes later. It starts behind the ears, spreads over the face, and then to the body. The small red spots quickly fuse into large blotchy areas closely resembling a large map. Strangely enough, it is in a way comforting when the rash eventually appears. Firstly knowing what is the matter with the child is a relief, and secondly the child almost always feels better at this point.

There is no special care after this point, other than sensible home nursing. If the eyes become sore and 'sticky', the child may be quite distressed on waking to find that he or she cannot open them and cannot therefore see. Bathe them gently with a clean cotton wool swab for each eye. One tablespoon of salt dissolved in hot water then cooled, will provide a suitable lotion. Sometimes the child may also be uncomfortable in full daylight if this is bright. Respect this, and create a comfortable level of light, at the same time ensuring that under such conditions there is no possibility of the child straining his or her eyes to read, or follow any similar activity.

There is usually no need to keep the child in bed during the day. Even when the child is at his or her most miserable, just before the rash appears, it is easier for mother and child, to make him or her comfortable in a family room. The child will feel less isolated, and can have his or her needs attended to, without too much running around by the parents. The general needs are extra fluids, good ventilation, extra bathing or sponging, and company.

It should be noted, that any other young children in the family, although they will probably develop measles also, could be offered gamma globulin, if the doctor recommends it. This is prepared from the blood of people who have manufactured the appropriate antibodies, and its introduction will cause an unprotected person to resist an attack of measles, or possibly only suffer a mild illness. It is very expensive, and in short supply, so would only be offered if there is some express need. For instance, if the child at risk, is very young, or already sick, or newly recovered from some illness. The complications of measles can be serious, even life threatening. Laryngitis, bronchitis, ear infections, diarrhoea, vomiting, conjunctivitis, or kidney infection, even measles meningitis has been recorded as a complication of measles. If the child's temperature rises suddenly after the initial fever has subsided, if the urine changes in colour, smell, or quantity, if the child has pain or stiffness in the limbs, or ceases to respond normally, call the doctor immediately. Early treatment can avoid permanent problems.

GERMAN MEASLES

Normally German measles is of a minor nature and one which most parents wish to have over and done with, in early childhood. As has been mentioned, the effects in unborn children of mothers contracting this disease in early pregnancy can be devastating. It is therefore vital that all young girls who reach puberty without acquiring immunity should be vaccinated. The symptoms are similar to those of measles, but less severe. The rash appears at the same time, and can be confused with measles, although it does not tend to fuse into patches. If there is any glandular swelling behind and below the ears, German measles may be confirmed.

Treatment once again, is sensible home nursing care, together with the extra tolerance often required when a child is unwell.

MUMPS

Again the first signs and symptoms of mumps are associated with the throat and head. There is usually stiffness and tenderness over the parotid gland area, around the angle of the jaw. The throat is probably very sore and food may be refused. Offer plenty of fruity drinks, lemon being particularly beneficial as this stimulates the salivary glands, causing saliva to flow and make the mouth more comfortable. Chewing gum also produces the same effect, and helps to prevent the jaw from becoming too stiff.

Mumps can be most uncomfortable for male adolescents and adults, at times affecting the testicles quite seriously, even causing sterility, although this is rare.

The incubation period is a long one, about 3 weeks, and the disease is relatively uncommon under 5 years. Adults may feel very ill indeed, however, and sympathy is well deserved, even though the victim usually presents a very amusing picture to friends and family. Deafness is a recognized complication and any doubts about affected hearing should be referred to the doctor. The recommended isolation period is 7 days after swellings disappear.

CHICKEN POX

Most children will experience an attack of chicken pox by the time they reach 10 years of age. It is thought that the same virus causes shingles in adults, and due to this, an adult sufferer from this disease may give a child chicken pox.

The incubation period is about 2 weeks, and patients are infectious for a day or so before the spots appear, until they have all become covered by dry crusty scabs.

The first sign is usually of a small number of spots, which quickly form purulent looking heads, which may break and become weepy. It is difficult for children not to scratch when the scabs develop, and application of calamine and/or frequent tepid baths, to which potassium permanganate or bicarbonate of soda has been added, helps to relieve irritation.

Some patients may be covered in many spots, others have only a very small number indeed. One of the most uncomfortable places is on the scalp, especially if the hair is thick, as the natural warmth causes more intense irritation. One effective way of applying calamine, is by using a very soft thick paint brush. The movement is soothing to the skin, the relief is quick to achieve, and the young patients really do enjoy it.

Head lice

Children from all sorts of home, and from all social categories are exposed to the risk of head lice. These determined parasites are no respector of person, and even tend to prefer a clean head or host. The female will lay her eggs on single hairs close to the head, often behind the ears, cementing them to each hair very firmly indeed. They can be seen clearly, once the observer knows what to look for. The lice are more difficult sometimes as they move away from the light, as the hair is parted. Once spotted however the treatment should be as immediate as practicable. These parasites can quickly pass from head to head, and lay many eggs. Solutions and shampoos are available from clinics and chemists. They are pleasant to use, and the instructions are simple to follow. Once an individual has been found to be suffering from head lice or nits (the eggs), the whole family should be advised to use the prescribed lotion or shampoo, as it is likely that others at home will be hosts, whether or not they have realized it.

Skin infections

SCABIES

Scabies is another parasitic infection. The female will lay her eggs in a small channel she makes by burrowing under the skin. Usually, warm tender places are chosen, such as between the fingers or toes. This is no longer a common infection and can be treated with Benzyl Benzoate. Refer to a doctor.

IMPETIGO

Impetigo is an unpleasant looking skin infection, which does spread at an alarming rate, given the opportunity. It looks like a scabby area, which 'weeps' when the scabs are disturbed, but does not heal as a normal wound would do. It used to be treated with Gentian Violet, but effective though it was, antibiotics are now used, either by direct application, or orally. The child should be isolated from others, until effectively treated, and toilet articles kept for separate use.

RINGWORM

Ringworm is caused by a fungus affecting the body in a variety of ways. It can be found on the skin, scalp, or nails. Ringworm on the body or limbs, appears as a red scaly circle with a pale centre. It is quite simple to diagnose and may be effectively treated with Whit-fields ointment, obtainable from the chemist.

Ringworm of the foot, commonly known as Athlete's Foot appears between the toes, first as a peeling 'soggy' area of skin, which can spread to the sole of the foot. It is almost unknown in parts of the world where shoes and socks are not worn, the fungus developing easily in warm, dark, moist conditions. Treatment is partly by special ointment and powder, partly by careful hygiene, and separate use of toilet articles, and partly by wearing open shoes, sandles, or 'flip-flops', whenever possible.

The popularity of training shoes as everyday wear, may tend to encourage this particlar form of ringworm, as the feet become hot, and there is little circulation of air. Young boys may need to be encouraged to change their socks daily!

Ringworm of the scalp is identified by small, round, bare patches on the head, where the hair around the edge has broken off. Where these stumps of hair can be seen, the area affected is still developing. This condition seems to be stimulated by some emotional stress, and treatment, although medically effective, must be linked to the possibility of emotional causes. This particular type of ringworm cannot be caught from another person. The treatment by cortisone results in new growth of hair in a few weeks. It is vital to reassure the patient on this matter, as sometimes large areas of the scalp can be affected, even the whole head.

Food poisoning

Food poisoning may be suspected when there is sudden abdominal pain, vomiting and diarrhoea. This can range from mild discomfort to serious pain, and sufficient loss of fluid, to necessitate hospital treatment. Very young children and babies can become dehydrated in a short time, and any child who is vomiting, and suffering from diarrhoea, must replace lost fluids by drinking at very frequent intervals.

Food poisoning usually affects more than one member of a family, or sometimes whole groups, who have attended the same function. Many cases of food poisoning are resolved by nature, but babies and young children require very careful observation, and the doctor will advise if the adult is concerned. If in doubt consult him.

Similar symptoms indicate an infection of the gastrointestinal tract. If this infection is active in the large intestine or bowel area, it can be confirmed by laboratory testing, and the diagnosis will be one of gastroenteritis. This term is often used loosely for a case of diarrhoea and vomiting, but is not correct unless the bacteria is present. Treatment is by antibiotics, but in the meantime it is vital that the baby or child maintains an adequate fluid intake, and that this fluid is retained. If there is any reluctance on the part of the patient, try different methods of presentation, straws, vegetable colouring, novelty ice cubes, fruit flavoured jellies, ice lollies, even going back to a feeding bottle for a very young child, can encourage the consumption of extra fluids.

A result of diminished fluid intake may be one of constipation. If this arises, it is not advisable to administer laxatives or even worse, purgatives. These may result in a satisfactory bowel action, but does not encourage the system to function independently, which is vital for healthy well being. It is very easy to become dependent on self-administered medication, in place of natural and efficient body functioning.

In the western world, where the average intake of roughage has been well below that required, for many years, there is a relatively high incidence of cancer of the colon. In less developed countries, where roughage represents a high proportion of the average diet, this particular disease is almost unknown. The appearance on the shelves of bran-based cereals in increasing varieties, reflects the growing awareness of the need for roughage in the western diet.

NURSING THE SICK CHILD

During normal healthy development, every child will expect to suffer some hiccoughs in the form of minor illnesses, most of which will be nursed at home. It is helpful to remember certain points.

Unless the illness is of a very minor nature, such as a cold, or a day or two of general malaise, it is advisable to contact the doctor, follow his or her advice, and keep him or her informed. Having said this the next priorities are those of extra nourishment, special care of the environment, treatment of boredom, tolerance of varying temperament, and most important of all plenty of TLC (tender, loving, care).

Nourishment in relation to diet is obviously very important, the appetite is likely to be affected, and certain foods are regularly more popular than others, for patients. For instance, soup, yogurt, ice-cream, eggs, instant whips, milk jellies, and fruit, are universally acceptable. Yogurt especially, is well tolerated, when other foods, even milk drinks, may be rejected by the stomach. It is of course very nourishing too. Soups likewise, can offer high nutritional content. A good one to start with is tomato. The food should always be presented in very small quantities. It is so much better to ask for a little more, than feel unable to face a large portion. The method of presentation can persuade or discourage a delicate appetite, and with a little imagination the whole experience can be most enjoyable, even exciting for the child. Small brown and white sandwiches cut with animal pastry cutters can produce brown cows and white sheep on a green field (a paper napkin), each 'eating' a handful of grass (cress or water cress). Watch adults sharing gingerbread men with children. They will obviously be making the decisions of 'head' or 'legs' first. Similarly duck shaped pasta swimming in the soup is quite fun. A menu can be worked out with the patient, once he or she is old enough to participate. This always seems to be a successful activity.

The patient may be happier with frequent small snacks, than the traditional meals, at traditional times. These do not need to be any less nourishing if carefully planned.

The environment should be clean, safe, and well-ventilated. If the child needs to stay in bed it is often possible to make some arrangements, downstairs or if in a flat or bungalow, in a different environment, for a large part of the day. This allows the bed, and room, to be aired and cleaned, and also offers a change in surroundings, and a sense of involvement with the rest of the family and the daily routine.

If the child is immobile, ensure that he or she has something of interest to watch, through a window is ideal. Television is useful, if used with discretion, as is the radio, record player or tape recorder. These may be used to complement human company, not to replace it. There should be safe access to a selection of suitable toys and books, remembering that regression during illness will usually indicate that such materials will need to be appropriate for a younger age group, than that usually favoured. Even adults when sick, will find it impossible to concentrate on a familiar category of material and may happily enjoy reading relatively undemanding literature, for instance, magazines instead of books. Children likewise will probably get a lot of pleasure from toys they have ignored for some time.

Chapter 9
Children and Families At Risk

Due to the very nature of today's technological world children are unavoidably exposed to risks every day of their lives. Clearly, it is the responsibility of the adults caring for children to minimize the risks whenever and wherever possible. Fortunately, most adults fulfil their role of guardian in a most effective and caring way.

Accidents are nearly always the result of unintentional carelessness, ignorance, or lapse in concentration on the part of the adult. It should be pointed out that the adult may often be other than the one responsible for the child. Accidents also happen as a result of nature: trees fall across roads, lightening strikes, hurricanes, avalanches and floods occur. There are, however, far too many children who suffer pain at the hands of those who are entrusted with the role of guardian. As most children are cared for by parents or step-parents, they form the largest number guilty of such practice. The pain suffered may be physical, social, emotional or even intellectual; it is usually a combination of more than one. As each area of development is interdependent, all 4 areas are commonly affected.

NON-ACCIDENTAL INJURY

It is the incidence of physical cause or non-accidental injury which has been afforded much attention through the media in recent years. It is naturally an emotive subject and merits front page coverage when severe cases are publicized. It is estimated that, nationally, about 8,000 children suffer some non-accidental injury each year. About one fifth of this number may suffer damage of a permanent and incurable nature, such as brain damage, paralysis or blindness. Any number from 100-400 may die as a result of physical violence or neglect.

These figures are horrific and any so-called civilized nation should be ashamed and concerned enough, to mount a comprehensive programme of prevention. Most of the programmes at present are initiated by voluntary bodies, and largely supported by charity.

There is no national education project aimed at preparation for parenthood. This role can no longer be left to develop naturally. The changing society economically and socially, makes parenting a much more complex and demanding exercise. Young parents frequently find themselves isolated when they need help most. Immediate family on whom they could rely are probably hundreds of miles away.

To substitute for this lack of support, in some areas, groups of young mothers have arranged meetings in each other's homes. More importantly, they have developed a network of people who may be facing similar problems and feel able to contact each other quite spontaneously when the need for support arises. Such groups, however, are relatively rare and need to be encouraged on a much wider basis, but without the intervention of statutory bodies, other than to facilitate such developments.

Statistics indicate, that children with certain historical criteria tend to be more at risk than others. Such criteria as low birth weight, prematurity, age of mother, standard/quality of housing, unwanted pregnancy, unwanted sex of child, marital relationships, financial security or lack of it, separation after birth of mother and child, all seem to be predisposing causes for subsequent child abuse. One of those which seems to have most effect is the quality of the parents' own experience (of parenting) during the vital early years. Abused children tend to become abusing parents, modelling their behaviour on the only model they know. Hence the term 'cycle of deprivation'. The next stage encountered, if education is not provided, and predisposing causes exist, could be positive signs of abuse. It is useful to know what to look for and how to come to the decision as to whether to seek further advice.

When young children are already in statutory care of some sort, it is easier to observe and record any disturbing signs, such as bruising or other small wounds. Before a child is determined to be officially 'at risk', however, he or she must be seen to be in danger.

Any child born subsequently to parents who have ill-treated or seriously neglected other children will automatically be termed 'at risk', as will other siblings living at home. If children have been taken into residential care under a court order, subsequent children can be removed from home shortly after birth.

VISIBLE SIGNS

Signs which should be recorded and reported:
1 Any new bruises, wounds, or marks on any part of the child.
2 Any notable change in movement, or obvious reluctance to take certain physical exercise.
3 Excuses made by children to avoid changing for physical education or swimming.
4 Absence by 'child at risk' not clearly explained.
5 'Story' of injury not matching the actual wounds or marks displayed.
Punching in the eye does not produce similar bruising to walking into a door, although the latter is a popular excuse. Cigarette burns are very distinctive, small, round wounds. Once they have been observed no other reason for such marks is acceptable.

Emotional abuse or neglect is much more difficult to detect or diagnose; consequently there must be many children who suffer in this way and never receive help. This treatment is almost impossible to prove in legal terms. The evidence is very subjective.

Specific examples

In over 90 % of all abused children there are visible signs, specific examples include:
1 Bruising around the mouth or injury to the frenulum or tongue, is rarely accidental, and all such injuries should be regarded as suspect.
2 Finger/thumb size bruising, matching the pattern of a grip or hold, either on the face or body. The child will display such signs as a result of being held down or shaken. Finger tip bruises are small and round or oval and cannot be felt when running hands over the skin area.

3 Unusual outline of an object used to hit a child, displayed by redness of skin in a defined pattern. The most common instruments used are fists, sticks and belts. The centre of the wound will remain white due to the blood being forced outward on impact and causing the capillary walls to burst.

4 Bite marks, unfortunately, have been diagnosed as administered by human beings. The pattern will be of two crescents separated at each side. The area defined will change from red to blue/black as bruising develops from haemorrhaging. There may be small wounds where a single tooth has broken the skin. The identity of the attacker can be proved through forensic examinations.

5 Scratches, although they can be quite ugly, can be caused by jealous siblings during vigorous play, or by the pet cat. It is difficult to differentiate if inexperienced, or if there is not a strong relationship with the mother/family. In the latter instance the 'story' attached to the scratches can be diagnosed, honest or suspect.

6 Scalds and burns. It is, once again, difficult to decide whether or not such incidents are truly accidental. It is the credibility of the history of the accident, matching of the wound to such history, and knowledge of the family which will combine to allay fears, or alert towards further investigation. Display of actual fear towards fire, or other hot objects should be noted with concern.

7 Swelling around joints resembling a sprain should be viewed with suspicion as this type of injury is rarely caused by natural accident in young children.

8 The signs of brain damage, probably the result of violent shaking, swinging by the legs or banging of the head, are, sleepiness, lack of eye coordination and signs of paralysis. This type of injury, contrary to popular belief, is the commonest cause of death from child abuse. It is probably the most difficult type for which to gather evidence which would be accepted in a court of law, unless the person responsible confesses.

Internal injury

Another category, that of internal injury is responsible for the second biggest number of child abuse deaths and, again, will not be reflected by visible bruising, although it is common to find other signs of abuse. The child will obviously be unwell, with a high temperature, malaise, probable vomiting and visible signs of being in pain. Clearly these symptoms are associated with many ailments and it is the overall family history and the familiarity with the total situation which is necessary to make the decision as to whether or not the case is suspect.

Unexplained deaths

Cot deaths or sudden infant deaths still remain largely unexplained. Proportionally, however, a larger number happen within families who present similar criteria to those who are termed 'at risk', than to families presenting no such criteria. There is difficulty in distinguishing between a cot death and suffocation, for the expert carrying out the post mortem examination.

There is knowledge of several children within families being suffocated before an accurate diagnosis was made. For example one child of an immigrant family appeared to have died in mysterious circumstances and it appeared to be a cot death. However, she was 2½ years old, older than could be accepted and her temperature was unusually low. Although impossible to prove, it was thought that the child had probably been smothered, as a younger sibling had also been 'found' dead a few weeks earlier under circumstances which could not be logically explained.

Drowning, unfortunately, is not always accidental. It is said, but again almost impossible to confirm, that children may be pushed into, or held under water. Efforts to rescue or revive may not always be maximized, reflecting at times a subconscious wish to remove a child, who presents problems beyond the coping level of individual parent/s.

Environmental factors

Environmental dwarfism or failure to thrive, is the result of lack of provision rather than the infliction of pain or abuse. These children do not present any detectable symptoms of disease, yet they do not grow and/or develop according to the norm, or within the range accepted as normal. In order to ascertain whether or not the rate of growth is satisfactory, measurements of height, weight and head circumference of all children thought to be 'at risk' should be recorded at regular intervals and records not only maintained, but interpreted professionally at similar regular intervals.

Obviously deviations from acceptable gains are easier to detect during the very early years of life, when such growth and development are rapid. Proportionally the child may be more representative of an earlier developmental stage. The limbs normally grow longer as the long bones grow rapidly, therefore, those which remain shorter than one would expect during early/middle childhood may never become part of a balanced, mature skeletal framework. Deprivation can be the cause. Food may be processed in an inefficient way, passing through the system too quickly, thus depriving the body of its nutritional needs. Stress can cause this to happen at any age, but the adult will probably suffer only occasionally in this way, whereas the child at risk may exist in a state of constant stress and be a victim of chronic diarrhoea. The appetite may be very good, even abnormally so. The emotionally deprived child will eat to console himself or herself and can put on too much weight, thus threatening healthy development, illustrating a link between emotional and physical progress.

CASE 1

Mary was a child privately fostered by her white unmarried mother. Mary's father was an African medical student so the child was a 'half caste'. The fostering broke down, due to unproved emotional and physical abuse by the unregistered 'foster' mother.

The reason for the problems encountered in providing evidence, were, that actions such as swatting with a newspaper to prevent a young child from sleeping, and forcing her to stand for long periods in the aisle of a cinema or in a corner, leave no discriminating physical marks. After various moves however, Mary found herself in residential care where the only word she spoke was 'more' and she ate all she could persuade the staff to give her. Her stomach became quite distended and almost reached her knees when sitting down.

Weight gain alone does not reflect healthy normal development. The other categories must progress at the same time and, although Mary gained weight, she did not play, speak, or make any social advances towards the staff. Happily, when placed in a stable family situation, a normal developmental pattern slowly established itself, although making relationships did remain a problem throughout childhood and may be so throughout life. The trust, which a child needs to feel in the adults caring for her, had not been established until too late for Mary to be able to adopt it as part of her basic personality. She may always distrust instinctively.

STAGES OF DEVELOPMENT

Trust

Erikson emphasizes the importance of trust in his first stage of development (Erikson 1967). He says that where the mother, or substitute, provides satisfactory care in every aspect the infant learns to trust his or her environment and lives with the security of firm predictability. As a direct result confidence develops and the child begins to experiment and explore physically, emotionally and socially. Obviously in this way learning takes place as well as the development of communication with the world, physical and personal.

According to Erikson, trust is necessary for these stages to be successfully negotiated in early infancy.

Independence

The next stage outlined by Erikson is that of emerging independence coming to terms with cooperation and authority. Success will be illustrated by clear self expression, desire to be independent without rejection of the adult within a relationship, and an acceptance of some authority figures as part of a happy existence. If control is unreasonable or inconsistent, such areas of development will be hindered or distorted.

Conscience

In early childhood a third stage is identified by the emergence of a primitive conscience. The child will display and feel guilt for deeds not approved by the adult model. Once again, if that model is over-dominant or inconsistent, the child will find it very difficult to act independently. He or she will resist making social advances and without the parental presence, may even be unable to make decisions in fear of making the 'wrong' one. This can be observed in Nursery or School when offering choices to children. Some become visibly confused and even upset by the challenge of decision-making. Similar problems will arise when parents 'talk' for their children, they feel totally unsupported when alone, and unable to express themselves adequately.

The three stages mentioned will normally take place during the first 4-5 years of life.

PROFESSIONAL INVOLVEMENT

One of the most obvious problems reflected in some of the recent serious cases of child abuse have been those of communication between parties professionally involved. It is, therefore, useful to look at some of those who commonly take a role in any case of child abuse or neglect. Nursery matrons, staff nurses, playgroup leaders and teachers, although very often the first to diagnose some problem, have no actual powers at all. They are, however, responsible for the child during the time in which the parent has entrusted them with care.

The observation skills developed during the training of nursery nurses are vital. Teachers and playgroup leaders do not have the benefit of such practice as part of their training or education. Doctors, nurses, psychiatrists, psychologists, health visitors and probation officers similarly have no specific powers in respect of child abuse or nonaccidental injury. They may, of course, be directly involved and able to produce acceptable evidence in their role as professionals.

Those who do have powers are police officers, social workers representing the Department of Social Services, and NSPCC Inspectors. They may all institute legal proceedings. For the police these will be of a criminal nature; for the remaining two categories, of a civil nature. Civil proceedings will normally be in respect of a child thought to be in need of care, control or protection. Through a Justice of the Peace, a Place of Safety Order may be obtained to remove a child judged to be in imminent danger. This order may be obtained if necessary at any time of the day or night.

FAMILIES AT RISK

Although it is true that no single social class will be exclusively linked with incidents of child abuse, those subjected to a greater degree of stress find their threshold of tolerance lower and, therefore, more likely to be threatened. The factors contributing to stress will be those affecting basic human needs. Love and security and freedom could probably provide the headings for all basic needs.

Parents living alone are frequently existing on a low income, in poor housing conditions, and may be emotionally and socially isolated. Consider the unmet needs here. Second marriages or common law unions both present possible problems. Second wives and subsequent children often have to budget extra carefully due to the father's financial responsibility towards his first wife and children. To alleviate this the second wife may be obliged to go out to work, which can understandably lead to fatigue and resentment. Consider the implications for the relationships involved. The common law union has obvious disadvantages due to the insecurity of the situation both emotionally and legally. It must be pointed out, however, that the Law is becoming more and more sympathetic towards 'injured' parties of common law unions. Some would say it is an advantage to have no legal obligations to stay together. On the one hand it means the couple really wish to be together and the voluntary element actually helps the relationship. On the other hand, one may feel entitled to leave without feeling any guilt or responsibility.

Parents who are below average intellectually will tend to hold jobs which are afforded little status or have no job at all. This causes the self image to be poor which, together with the attendant stress factors of such an existence, causes an unstable and unpredictable environment for the whole family unit.

CULTURAL DIFFERENCES

Other cultures may have their own method of bringing up their children and their patterns of discipline and punishment can cause unreasonable criticism to be levelled against them. It is not so very long ago that young children went to work down the mines, in factories and as domestic servants in this country. It is also not so very long ago that a child could be hanged for stealing a loaf of bread.

It is reasonable that all elements of a human society will not approach some problems within that society in a similar way. The ability to move from one culture to another so easily means that the varying stages of development are thrown together and the inevitable conflict is found in the process of each having to coexist with the other.

This can be seen particularly when large numbers of immigrants settle in their new country forming sizeable communities. Those representing law, order and control will be predominantly indigenous and very unlikely to be familiar with other ways of social control. Families who have been used to exercising a high degree of authority over their children find this hard in the new environment, and they are challenged by their young. These young people then challenge the other authority figures within schools and the police service. Without respect for any form of authority, the result can be widespread public disorder as seen in Toxteth, Brixton and Bristol in late 1981.

SEVERITY OF PUNISHMENT

The question must be raised as to whether physical punishment is ever justified. If so, by whom should it be administered and where does abuse begin? Teachers are most reluctant to use such methods to achieve control no matter how severely provoked by bad, even violent, behaviour. They are open to prosecution by the 'victim' however mild the action.

It is just as difficult to judge whether or not a parent has reasonably chastised his or her own child. Many older people may say 'Well, my father beat me regularly and it never did me any harm.' There is no proof either way, but such actions may well be open to prosecution today.

POSSIBLE PROTECTION

Refuges

Within families where children are at risk, it is likely that the mother, or even in rare cases the father, is also at risk. Violence towards young children is bizarre and totally incongruent with normal behaviour. Those who can abuse children may also abuse others who have little defence. Mothers present such targets for the distorted personalities. So widespread is. such practice that places of refuge have been set up in various parts of the country, where women and children may go and be guaranteed safety. Erin Pizzey founded the first refuge in Chiswick, since then hundreds of women and children have been harboured and protected from violent abusive men.

There are those who present the argument that some women actually enjoy being physically ill-treated, otherwise they would not stay. This is a ridiculous statement—where can they go? In most cases they and their children cannot be taken in by members of the family, and there is no recognized statutory place of safety.

The refuges which do exist are in no way attractive enough to persuade women to leave home unless the situation they are in is absolutely impossible and the women feel themselves and their children to be in physical danger. They are usually overcrowded, causing lack of privacy, often in 'run-down' areas and sparsely furnished. The limited funds available from statutory and voluntary sources have to be spread thinly due to the policy strongly held, of never turning away any mother and children in need of protection. Added to this, the very real fear of being found and threatened further, may mean that the family is obliged to spend most of the time in the house. This obviously leads to stress and tension between families and children, who are already suffering quite acutely from such pressures.

These places of refuge do offer a 'first aid' treatment but such a remedy is obviously not satisfactory on a long-term basis, and some attempts have been made to provide for longer term programmes. It has to be accepted that many cases of serious family problems will only be diagnosed through actual injury to a child or children. Therefore, it is from this point in time, that consideration will be directed.

Care orders

The urgent action to be taken is that of immediate protection against the possibility of further injury. This usually means admitting the child to hospital, a procedure not often resisted by a parent who will see this as an acceptable decision. If the parent does not agree to such a move, then in order to protect the child a Place of Safety Order may be sought. Anyone may make such application to a Magistrate for a child to be removed and kept in a place of safety for up to 28 days. The police can take action without making such an application, but the child may only be detained for a period of up to 8 days.

An interim care order will commit a child to the care of the Local Authority for a period of up to 28 days. A Juvenile Court will make such an order.

In cases of suspected child abuse, care orders are much more likely to be taken than criminal proceedings. When an order has been processed there will be considerable effort put in by various professionals to furnish a comprehensive report. Contributions to such a document may include a health visitor, a general practitioner, a social worker, the police or an NSPCC Officer, and the officer in charge of a Nursery. Obviously not all of these would always be involved. As a result of this report and its analysis and interpretation, further orders may be made.

The care order transfers to the local authority the legal parental rights. The authority decides where the children shall live and may even decide to allow them home under guidance or supervision. Sometimes the children will be placed in community homes or foster homes and cases should be reviewed every 6 months. If when reviews take place the order is renewed, the order can continue to be effective until the eighteenth birthday. The authority, the parent or guardian, or the young person may apply for an order to be revoked. This can be approved or a supervision order made instead.

A supervision order can last up to 3 years and it is the duty of the social worker, usually appointed, to maintain effective links with the family, building up a relationship conducive towards solving some of the problems within the family unit.

Parental recognizances which require the guardian to exercise proper care and control may be taken out only with the consent of the parent. They may be conditional upon a certain sum of money being named and to be effective up to 3 years. This would probably operate in a similar way to bail. These orders are rarely applied. In a similar way, hospital orders may be taken out when necessary to ensure proper care after discharge.

Appeals against any orders may be made, also against refusals to discharge orders. Notice of such action must be made within 21 days by, or on behalf of, the Child Legal Aid and is available subject to the usual conditions.

RE-ESTABLISHING THE FAMILY UNIT

After legal procedures have been negotiated, the real work towards establishing a happy, stable and independent family unit will begin. Effort to achieve totally satisfactory results requires much and there remain far too many children 'in care' due to the failure of the professional team. The word 'failure' to achieve the desired result may seem aimed in a critical sense towards the social worker. In reality, any steps successfully made towards improvement within the family situation are small battles won, even though the war may eventually be lost. The effort must always be made.

Setting objectives

One way in which help may be planned is by setting objectives or goals. Success can then be measured by matching achievement against such predetermined targets. Objectives need to be clearly defined and initially they need to be easily obtainable. They should ideally be negotiated between professional and client. Such practice will prevent the worker becoming the controlling, probably patronizing figure, representing authority, and any progress will be seen as shared success. Sometimes a sensible and realistic routine worked out between both parties can alleviate some of the pressure caused by physical and emotional demands overtaking the competence level of the mother as she sees it.

Priorities need to be established. Small children must have love, security and freedom. Love is frequently strong, though poorly expressed due to other pressures. Security is often a struggle and simple, commonsense budgeting does not come naturally to all people. If they have never been taught by their own parents how to manage available money in a practical way, they learn through costly trial and error.

Budgeting

Budget objectives could involve:

1 Defining precisely income, and regular unavoidable outgoings.
2 Assessing the extent to which expenditure exceeds income each week.
3 Reducing this to a 'break even' state with help from the social worker or other trusted person.
4 Looking carefully at items which are 'impulse' buys.
5 Making a shopping list and sticking to it.
6 Learning to produce two new 'budget' meals each week.
7 Setting aside a cupboard or shelf and buy something every shopping trip to add to this store.
8 Starting to save, with 10p a day to begin with and leaving the money for an agreed length of time.
9 Deciding at which point in the programme you deserve a reward. Decide on the reward, and award it at the appropriate time. Share your success.
10 Counting the successes and carrying on, if you 'fail' at any point. The old saying 'Look after the pennies and the pounds will take care of themselves' does make sense.

Behavioural responses

If a parent was regularly resorting to even moderate physical punishment, a similar set of objectives could be written. The starting point may be a record of what specific actions on the part of the child cause such a response from the parent. The exercise of keeping such a record will not only draw the attention of the parent to each incident, even when alone and unsupervised, but also will illustrate how inconsistencies can exist in the parent's repsonses. I would recommend that any parent who is concerned in any way about an inability to handle their children, without resorting to physical means, should have access to such documents through health visitors, or even Libraries and Social Security Offices. A local number where help and support is available could be added.

LONG-TERM HOPE

If, hopefully, there is success in eliminating the physical abuse within a family unit, it cannot be assumed that a 'cure' has been effected and everyone will live happily forever after. This assumption can itself be a contributory cause towards a further situation of risk. The first situation arose from certain predisposing causes which may not necessarily have been removed. The parent figures may still present personality disorders, still be subjected to various stress factors, and if educationally subnormal will inevitably remain so. The child may be healed physically but not emotionally, a situation which tends to be afforded less attention.

The parents may not have been introduced in an effective way to alternative methods of care and control. Local staffing levels will normally preclude an ideal programme of family support for a recommended period.

There is no easy answer to diagnosed cases of child or family abuse. All members of the affected unit are involved, and may all need some sort of support, to a greater or lesser degree. Such support would probably need to be of a prolonged nature and administered by specially developed and trained personnel. Such resources are in short supply. Although a preventive programme would be demanding, there are more skilled 'amateur' personnel available who could help to prevent, than there are to cure. Such personnel include experienced parents within the community, e.g. Parents Anonymous. There are more 'good models' than 'bad'.

Chapter 10
Planning Group Activities

One of the challenges encountered by any newcomer to the world of child care is that of building up, in a short time, an adequate fund of ideas for group activities. To give the new practitioner a small repertoire, this section will cover a representative range of activities found in any good curriculum together with examples of related ideas.

It is not commonly accepted that very young children will follow the familiar categories of subjects, but for the purpose of presenting easily identifiable units, the traditional subjects will be used, as planning is facilitated in this way.

The nursery nurse should become involved in the learning activities followed by the children. Genuine interest should be displayed and similarly delight in achievement, at the same time sensing disappointment and recognising problems. The nursery nurse's attitude should be as natural as possible, certainly avoiding using a 'special' voice either talking down or sweetly softening the tone.

DRAMA

Intelligent observation of children will confirm that much of their time is spent both in solitary and cooperative dramatic or role play. This can be encouraged by the provision of dressing-up clothes, home corners, and other specific 'sets', e.g. hairdressing or shop corners. Home play is particularly interesting if it can be unobtrusively observed (Fig. 10.1). Most of the time it is sufficient to enable and facilitate rather than organise and direct. The spontaneity is of more value than a predetermined scenario planned by adults.

It is on some occasions necessary to present some sort of 'production' for parents, who welcome the involvement. Such activities usually take place at the end of a term or around the date of some specific holiday or festival. Music is usually part of the presentation

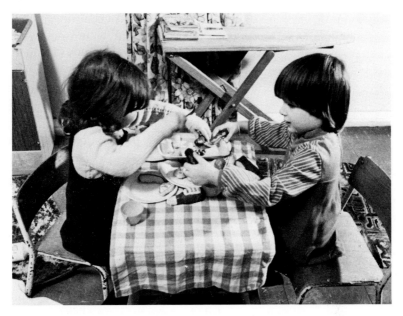

Fig. 10.1 Role playing can reflect a true home situation or uncover new skills.

and very young children will enjoy the secrecy of preparation and rehearsals, together with the excitement of the performance.

When observing children engaged in role play avoid trying to interpret their words and behaviour too analytically. It is easy to make presumptions, but children who seriously smack a doll or teddy bear are most unlikely to be communicating a case of child abuse, or dangerous aspirations to power!

READING

Children must master the task of reading as early as possible as without such an ability all other activities at school may be affected. It is accepted that all learning tends to be more readily and successfully encountered when young. The children of immigrant families become familiar with a second language much more easily than their parents, even accepting that they may be surrounded by that language at school. When learning to drive, it is said that 1 hour of instruction is required for every year of life.

It should also be appreciated that learned habits are difficult to change, and therefore patterns established early in life ought to be of the most efficient and useful nature. Those who act as the facilitators, providers, enablers, instructors or models, through which learning is acquired, carry considerable responsibility.

Reading and understanding are not always necessarily congruent skills. The ability to interpret a collection of letters into a language component is one skill, the ability to understand its meaning and to be able to use it spontaneously in an appropriate way, is another. *Spruit, pinfold* and *gloze* are not difficult to read, but using them appropriately demands further knowledge.

Stages in learning

The first step in the development of what is a complex and unnatural skill is the adequate acquisition and development of language. Next is the acquaintance with the printed word. This is a whole new world through which the mind may go beyond individual experience, into those of reality and fantasy recorded for the purpose of sharing. The written word is a vehicle of release, from the limitations set by personal experience. It should be presented to the young child as a vehicle of excitement not as a chore. As a tool which can be mastered and used with great skill and craftsmanship by those who practise and persevere. Perseverance is an attribute displayed by young children quite voluntarily in many types of unsupervised play. The skill of teaching children to read is closely linked to the skill of harnessing this perseverance. To do this, the whole exercise must be of relevant use to the child and he or she must appreciate this. At times he or she will be quite happy to use fun as legitimate relevance, e.g. using jokes as vehicles for learning to read, and activities leading to the skill of reading can often explore this side of learning situations. To read, it is necessary to recognize symbols, and combinations of symbols, and transfer them into appropriate sounds. This ability will become automatic, but to do so requires much practice.

Symbols and patterns

First of all, games can be made to encourage careful observation of symbols and patterns. Playing cards provide a useful source of good quality pictures often in sets of four. These can be used in the following ways.

1   Distribute the cards at random between the children and ask them to find their twin, triplet, or quadruplet. Match the cards to a number in the group. This activity will give rise to some interesting comparative language.

2   Stick one set of pictures onto a large card and ask the child to cover each card with a card which will match exactly. Such descriptive language as 'exactly the same', 'every detail', 'slight difference', 'precisely' and 'accurate' can be introduced. It is sometimes useful to ask why a card is unlike another as this requires more explanation, especially if the adult finds it 'difficult' to understand at first.

3   Distribute the cards and keep a set. Describe a picture verbally and the child who successfully identifies a card in his or her hand can hand it over. The first to achieve an empty hand can win, or takes over the job of description. This game can obviously be as simple or sophisticated as required.

4   Turn the cards face downwards on a large flat surface and taking it in turns, 'find' a matching pair. Games such as these develop the skills of discrimination, memory and concentration.

5   Bingo may be played with picture cards, ordinary playing cards, or simple words, as can most of the games already mentioned. The child will need to know the sounds that individual letters represent and 'I spy' using a written symbol is helpful. Hold a card with a single letter or useful combination such as 'ch' and pause just before making the sound. This will hopefully attract the attention of the children when both the sound and symbol can be presented simultaneously.

Although not universally recommended for very young children as an activity they really do enjoy chanting and ritual. This can be harnessed into a useful vehicle for the more tedious categories of learning. Such as sounds of the alphabet, months of the year, and the old demon, times tables. There are few adults who do not rely on such memories at times. In answer to questions such as 'How many days in the month of June?', or, '7 × 8?', most will rely on very early rote learning or chanting of rhymes and sequences. How else does one use a dictionary or telephone directory in an efficient manner? It cannot be denied that some very early rote learning, when it can still be fun, will undoubtedly prove useful later in life.

WRITING

Writing which develops into a highly individual trade mark for each person, has its roots in a system which with few small differences is very similar. The system involves each person learning in an identical manner to a prescribed pattern.

Children will learn to hold a writing tool, graduating from a thick crayon, or chalk, pencil or brush, to a refined implement in each category. This skill is obviously closely linked to reading and once a child realizes that he or she can have some control over the written word, creativity is born. It is thought by some experts that spelling and punctuation are less important than content. To reach a high level of competence in any activity it is necessary to discipline oneself to follow rules. Once these are mastered creativity will emerge, and in principle this applies to literacy just as to any other skill even football. There are always rules.

Start the child by encouraging him or her to hold a writing or drawing implement in the accepted way, not in a fist hold. Provide plenty of materials: paper, chalkboard, special wall panels, glass, mirrors and pavements. These can all be used, but may not all be appropriate in every situation.

As well as free expression help the child to follow patterns which develop the skill of forming curves and loops. Teach him or her to progress from left to right, not always easy for the left hander. Establish the habit of starting at the top of the page making rows of patterns, and incorporate many of the movements necessary to form written letters.

When the child begins to copy his or her name and other words, watch the way in which the letters are formed. They may well look perfect when the task is completed, but the actual formation may well be inefficient for future conversion to cursive or 'joined up' writing. For instance, it is common for 'a' to be made by drawing a circle 'O' and attaching a stick. Likewise an 'm' is made with the addition of an 'l' = 'm'.

It is very difficult for reasons already mentioned to 'undo' established habits. Writing must be taught in a specific way, every individual will develop his or her own unique style later in life, and it is surprising how soon the unique characteristics emerge. Sometimes it is useful to accompany the actual drawing of letters with a verbal commentary. This aid to concentration whilst engaged on a task is familiar at any age, even adults can be heard 'talking' to themselves whilst concentrating on a very demanding job.

Special care and attention should be paid to left handed children. They have specific problems such as the covering of that which they have already written. This means that they often have to turn the paper sideways or 'loop' their arm and hand over the top of the writing line. All right handed people should experiment in order to appreciate the problems encountered by left handers. One method they use is to change the position of paper and writing hand constantly during one page of script. The result is that the finished page may appear to have been written by different people, it certainly looks untidy and lacks regular patterning. It may however be the best that a left hander can produce having developed his or her own method of overcoming problems, in the absence of a left hander to guide him or her, during the early years of using implements for writing. These children also find it difficult at times to take dictated notes especially at speed. Remember many of the movements are for them 'backwards'.

ARITHMETIC

Arithmetic is described as the 'science of numbers', and as the 'art of reckoning' by figures. So, officially it is seen both as an art and a science. Whatever an individual's interpretation, the manipulation of figures has always seemed to present the student, from an early age, with more challenge than any other area of study. Maybe it is the totality of being right or wrong, that threatens. There is no degree of accuracy which is acceptable and the solution to a problem can be very elusive. It will help children to approach number work with confidence if their early experiences are positive and enjoyable.

If no-one hints that numbers can be hard to master then children will not anticipate problems.

Language of comparison will be part of every day use. Words such as big, bigger, biggest, more, less, higher, lower, will form part of natural conversation, and should be associated with their real meaning.

Counting often becomes a meaningless chant, and parents may be sure that counting the stairs means that the understanding of numbers is directly related. Real understanding, however, means knowing all about a number. Take 'five' for example. The properties which should be appreciated are:

1   That its property remains constant, always representing five, whether people, oranges, pence or anything else.

2   That five may be made up of $2 + 2 + 1$, $3 + 1 + 1$, $1 + 1 + 2 + 1$, $1 + 1 + 1 + 1 + 1$, $4 + 1$, $3 + 2$, and 5. These can be presented in a visual way using a variety of units.

3   Numbers relate to collective nouns. For example, two bananas, two apples, and one plum, will make a set of five fruits. Encourage the children to look for common properties to determine the classification label for a set. For example, a collection of articles from a handbag will form a 'set found in a handbag'. This attribute is common to them all.

Offer the children various collections of items and ask them to sort them out into different boxes or tins. Find out what criteria have been used and discuss the logic with the children. Ask the children to sort themselves into sets. This will involve discussion, decision-making, and execution of an activity, related to a decision made. A complex set of skills.

4   Playing games using dice provides practice in recognizing a number of dots, relating it to the spoken word, and finally to a number of moves. Either the familiar or home made games can be played. In order to reverse the skill, the dice can display symbols or the written word.

Make basic mathematical language and processes part of everyday life. Include time, speed, weight, volume, length, and all such concepts in a natural and practical manner.

MUSIC

Music is an international language. Through it we can communicate the whole gamut of human emotions without any specific words being used. It crosses cultural boundaries without losing cultural identity and it crosses generations with effective communication, even though little appreciation is often expressed, by each, of the others music. Music brings people together especially in times of emotional upheaval, pleasant or unpleasant. Special types of music are composed in times of war, and in times of national well-being, as in the sixties when the Beatles and 'Flower people' reflected a sense of euphoria. All categories of intellect respond to, and enjoy music. Severely handicapped people are stimulated by music and respond by appropriate physical movements. Intelligent people also respond to a wide range of music. It is a vital part of life, every life.

Due to the fact that very few of the people qualifying to work with young children are able to read music or play an instrument it is necessary to use other tools. There is certainly no shortage of choice; records, tape recorders, and video recorders can provide an adequate and varied selection of musical activities at the push of a button or flick of a switch.

In some ways this can be an advantage, the adult can join in with the children, can be mobile and can explore a wider variety of activities. New games, songs, and poems can be learned together. It is unnecessary, even inadvisable to segregate music for very young children into a defined period during the day. It can, and should, be part of many other activities:

1   The adults should sing to young children, as well as talk to them from the moment they are born. It does not matter about being in key or hitting the notes accurately, it is an emotional, social stimulation not an academic exercise. Sing whilst out for a walk, whilst bathing the children, whilst going about everyday tasks and chores. The presence of constant radio music as background is not a substitute.

2   Use the radio. There are some excellent programmes linking music and physical activity, and dramatic play. These can be recorded and used at will, and are very often suitable for use at home for mother, nanny and child.

3 Play 'ring' games with the children, and make the effort to learn a selection, thoroughly.

4 Record short pieces of music which will illustrate parts of a familiar story, and pause during the tale to emphasize the chosen part in a musical way. The children can be introduced to light classical music in this way.

5 Use brass band music for marching. Encourage the children to listen and follow the beat. Ever better take them to watch soldiers marching if this can be done safely. Allow them to observe the best model.

6 Share percussion instruments between the children, but plan precisely how they are to be used. Too often there is simply a general confusion of sound, drowning the music, and a total lack of direction.

It is a mistake to assume that children need total freedom of expression at all times. This is unrealistic and divorced from life itself, where total freedom for the individual causes restrictions for others. It is the duty of the adult to prepare children for the next stage of development, and for successful social interaction. Planning, structure, and discipline all have their place in early childhood education.

PHYSICAL EDUCATION

Physical education may be observed when children are pulled to their feet during the latter part of their first year of life. Children do not learn to walk automatically, they are encouraged to imitate the adult model. Such education begins much earlier when the baby kicks in his or her bath, reaches out for a toy, achieves some form of motor ability, and coordinates eye and hand, to select and take hold, of some small object. Fortunately this category of development is a pleasurable experience for most children. They have a natural drive to experiment and test the limitation of their own bodies. It is up to the adult to ensure that their environment is safe, yet challenging. Equipment, i.e. climbing apparatus, wheeled toys, should be kept in good repair, and used sensibly. Younger children should rely on their own judgement, rather than attempting to imitate older friends or siblings. To do this, it is necessary to be well acquainted with normal child development, and also acquainted with the individual child, his or her skills and weaknesses, both physical and emotional. It is not always the superior physical specimen who displays the higher level of ability. Achievement depends on a set of general abilities, rather than on any specific one.

To encourage physical development, it is useful to remember the principle that the earlier the learning, the easier will be the effectiveness. To develop their physical education:

1 Always allow babies a period of time each day without the restriction of clothing. Make sure he or she is in a safe place, free from draughts, and enable him or her to experience all body movements. This will give the baby considerable pleasure.

2 Introduce the young baby to water, as an environment in which he or she may learn to survive happily, acquiring the vital skills for a life-time. A bath at home filled with warm water is sufficient for the baby to practise and even to learn to swim. Many pools now provide a **shallow area** for toddlers, and plan sessions for them and their mothers. *Never* leave a child unsupervised in water, however shallow, and for however short a period of time. It can lead to the most tragic and yet most preventable of accidents.

3 Set up short 'obstacle courses' for children according to their age and ability. Make sure that the tasks present a challenge, yet remain safe. Introduce an element of bravery if possible, such as a balancing walk, just high enough to be daring, or a tunnel long enough to become dark in the middle.

4 Climbing is almost always difficult for a child to resist, and therefore any natural ascents should be tried and well-tested before being placed on the permissible list. Even with children of 7 or 8 years of age it is a good idea to mark a point beyond which climbing is forbidden, if necessary.

5 Provide wheeled toys both of the push and pull along type, and riding variety. The skill of manoeuvering and anticipating problems is developed, together with the pleasure of controlling faster movements than can be experienced on foot. Basic road safety can be simulated by using prams, tricycles, and imitation roads and crossings.

6 Practise body control by games which demand change of movement on a given signal. Ask the children to skip or hop around the room, for instance, change direction on a signal and 'freeze' in another. Two signals will be sufficient for most groups and the variety of movement which can be introduced and practised is greater than might first be imagined.

7 Introduce ball skills starting with balloons and inflatable beach balls, followed by large soft rubber or plastic balls. For 7- to 8-year-olds table tennis, tennis or other similar balls can be used, but avoiding hockey, and hard cricket balls.

8 By the age of 7 or 8 children will understand and appreciate the need for, and value of, rules. It is helpful to guide them in the use of rules and respect for the role of the referee.

GEOGRAPHY

Geography begins with knowledge and awareness of the immediate, and then the widening environment. The concept of distance and size develops gradually and it is difficult to estimate when one can expect these to be established. There are some levels which still present problems to the educated and mature mind. Light years, for instance, and the speed of space travel, are difficult to relate to most adults' experiences. If we are seeing constellations as they were years ago, and if we were able to perceive detail, would any life observed be younger than now, or extinct? What is now?

Geography for the toddler extends to the boundaries of his or her everyday life. Places visited on holiday will not be associated with home by any concept of distance. The story of a journey will give a child some idea of how far. But what does a 'long way' mean to him or her? Even a toddler, however, may appreciate a 'map' of his or her environment.

1 Make a plan of one room, one floor, the garden, a familiar short walk, a ride in the car. The bare details can be prepared and the personal features added by the child. This introduces the child to the concept of a 'bird's eye' view, the first step in a useful skill during later life.

2 Make a map of the roads within a radius of half a mile or so. Take the child and the map out and trace the journey using the small 'footprint' stamp, available from stationers.

3   Using holidays or countries of origin of other children, or food, point out and mark locations on a world map. Personalize these with self portraits by the children, attached by threads, and by labels taken from the appropriate foods.

4   Introduce the children to the concept of different languages. There are simple songs which can be learned quite easily. Even better, invite people of different nationalities to come and meet the children, dressed if appropriate in their familiar dress.

5   Try having a regular time when either a French or German person will communicate in his or her language. The children will 'pick up' some of the language. The accent will be good, and if the pattern could be continued, the benefits accrued towards the acquired skill of a second language would be enormous.

6   Introduce children to foods from other countries, probably cooking some simple dishes yourself. Relate these to the world map, but never **expect** the children to demonstrate such knowledge. The aim really, is to sow the seeds for later learning. The tools for such learning must be part of life at an early age.

7   Try to arrange visits to types of environment unfamiliar to the child: sea, harbour, river, reservoir, waterfall, brook, and pond are fairly easy to identify.

8   Go to the zoo and match animals with country of origin, explaining why certain classes and types of animal, birds or insects may thrive successfully in certain climates and terrain.

HISTORY

History starts with yesterday, if not sooner, and the child needs first of all to begin to appreciate the concept of time. The immediate past is real to the child almost as soon as he or she can communicate his or her desires; needs can only be expressed verbally by relating to past experience.

Children see themselves in time, when stories about their earlier lives are irresistible. Just as with adults, it is difficult or impossible for them to imagine 'not being' and on seeing a photograph of parents on their wedding day will frequently ask 'Where am I'?

Maybe there are links with the common faith in an after-life. It is unacceptable to conceive the idea of 'not being'.

Concrete props are the best method of introducing the idea of 'old' and 'past'.

1   Ask the children to bring the oldest item of clothing belonging to them, to nursery or school. It will be interesting to compare the sizes of clothing, and present stature, especially if some baby clothes arrive. It can be discussed whether time always reflects growth, and what may happen in other ways to indicate age.

2   Living and dead things will illustrate the concept of a natural life span. Leaves in Autumn, seashells, flowers, pets, are linked to life and death.

Sometimes a child will experience the loss of a pet or elderly relative. It is presumptuous to assume that a child may be helped or taught to understand death. It is still one of the mysteries of life itself. The role of the caring adult is to prepare children for the inevitability of death, and to support them through any direct experience. It must be remembered that human beings of any age will allow themselves to assimilate emotionally only that with which they feel able to cope. It is a gradual process of grief, that total acceptance of loss is taken in stages. It is necessary to consider these thoughts, because history is essentially made up of people who are no more, together with their associated artefacts.

3   Photographs of children together with those of immediate relatives can be displayed in a 'family tree' pattern. If it is not possible to obtain photographs especially of great grandparents, the children can draw their own, often discussing what they may have looked like. They will also enjoy, and develop a better concept of time, if they draw the house and the road or shops, which may have been part of the environment of the great grandparents.

4   The programmes for schools on television often transmit short documentaries, plays, and stories, depicting life in a bygone era. The immediate past relating to one generation's span, can be linked to their parents' childhoods, and direct questioning can 'bring to life' such history.

5   Invite an old person, who is alert and communicative to come and tell the children about his or her own early life or schooldays. This is particularly successful if presented in narrative form.

6   Try to collect some items which illustrate a comparison between old and new. These can be displayed in pairs with labels offering brief details such as: 'This is a new hot water bottle', 'This is a very old bed warmer'. Books, postcards, ornaments, and toys can be contributed for an 'old and new' display.

7   Take the children, in very small groups, ideally not more than four to each responsible adult, to local places of interest. There are many accessible locations and in these days of constant car travel, it is surprising how little many adults know about the history of their own immediate area. Much can be learned by the adults, when planning and participating in activities for young children.

BIOLOGY

Two main areas, animal and human biology, and plant biology, will be discussed. These come under the categories fauna and flora.

Fauna

Children are naturally curious about their own bodies, they are interested in their sexual differences and their basic functioning. They will also be openly curious about physical deviations from the norm, and it is at this very early age, that understanding and tolerance of those mentally or physically disabled, may be born. Young children will accept and relate to these disabled or handicapped people without restraint. It is the adults who usually have the problems. Therefore all the more reason to facilitate integration in early education, when and where this is appropriate.

1   Through keeping pets, children will become familiar with the functions of eating and eliminating, and will relate those to themselves. They may also be fortunate enough to observe and participate in the reproduction cycle. They will be able to appreciate 'birth', as miniature replicas of the parent, as hairless helpless babies, and by hatching from eggs, bird or fish variety. There may be some reference to the fact that a male and female of a species is required to

produce offspring, but it is only necessary to make such reference in passing. Apart from any other reason, too many children now come from one parent families, and the assumption that there should be two parents, should never be made. The children in question cannot be expected to discriminate between biological functioning and their present situation.

2   Through caring for pets, which are dependent, children will learn to be responsible, gentle, and sensitive to others' needs. They will experience the sharing of pleasure and amusement, a very valuable social and emotional activity for human beings. Think how different it is, to watch or listen, to a sad or funny play or programme alone, or with someone sympathetic to similar set of emotions as oneself. Which would you choose to do? Through sharing the ups and downs of everyday life with children, their ability to cope and hopefully their sense of humour is developed. Both are essential tools for life.

3   There will be plenty of occasions on which minor accidents will be experienced by the children. They are usually fascinated by injury, and similarly by any loss of blood. Grasp the opportunity to reduce or eliminate any distress caused by the sight of blood. Using a microscope encourage the children to look at a drop spreading it evenly across a glass slide. They will be amazed at what they see. Talk about how healing takes place.

4   Take a drop of water from a pond, and focus under a microscope, the results are always amazing and fascinating. There is no risk of disappointment. Microscopes, the more powerful the better, should always be available for young children to use under supervision. Simpler instruments can be permanently on display together with a selection of specimens, which may be changed regularly.

5   Arrange to watch some of the programmes designed to educate young children about themselves, their bodies, and their abilities and the need to take responsibility for their own well-being. Start at a very young age to inform seriously about the dangers of smoking, eating foods containing suger, and the uselessness of 'junk' foods in terms of nutritional value, imagination and crudeness of flavour. Use heroes and heroines if necessary to present good models of health and well-being. Stress the mental alertness which is associated with health, and relate this to a high level of awareness in traffic, and when negotiating physical hazards.

6   When talking about positive health, point out the inevitability of small inconveniences such as coughs, colds, chickenpox, and minor accidents. At the same time, and in an atmosphere without stress or threat, e.g. when the children are healthy and fit, introduce the concept of injury or illness requiring hospital treatment.

A nurse or doctor may be happy to come and talk to the children, the former could wear her or his uniform. Uniforms often tend to dehumanize people, and an introduction in a familiar environment can only serve to allay any future apprehension.

It is less constructive to pretend that things 'will not hurt', when it is likely to prove untrue. There are many times in life when people are unavoidably hurt, physically and emotionally. Obviously the aim of the caring adult is always to protect the child. Protection is not always the most realistic preparation for life. Do point out to children that there will be occasions on which there will be hurt, there will be unhappiness, tears and suffering. Point out also, that those who love him or her, will be there to share and support, until the time for laughter returns. Anyone who has experienced situations in which children are found in pain or distress, will confirm that during these times there is often an opportunity to share a smile even though in objective terms things may appear temporarily without humour.

Coping with emotions is as relevant a skill as coping with physical challenges. Encourage children to help each other, as well as to know how to receive help. There are many adults who are unable to accept graciously either help, compliments, thanks, or advice.

Flora

It is impossible to come to terms with or appreciate the environment, without getting to know some of the living things found there.

1   All children will identify a flower or tree. What may be more confusing are types of these, and identification can be encouraged by collecting, and naming, pressed leaves and flowers, and using collectors, or 'I-spy' books.

2   Many vegetables and flowers, even fruits, can be grown quickly, with progress observed and recorded by the children. There is something very special about picking home grown radishes, brushing off the soil and crunching the 'hot' flesh of the root.

Plants, flowers and vegetables may be grown indoors. A large pot will accommodate a potato tuber, a runner bean plant, a broad bean plant, a strawberry plant, or a dwarf pea plant easily. It makes a change from the familiar plants usually found indoors, and allows children to see how the vegetables on their plates develop in the field or market garden.

3   Collect seeds of all types and discuss how they find their way to places where they can settle and grow into new plants. Experiment with a variety of environments to discover the most suitable for initial growth. Relate the required criteria to the human body, e.g. food, air, light, water and care.

4   Use the engine as an analogy for animal and plant survival. Each needs fuel as food, and the quality of this relates to the quality of growth or performance. If one's body is seen in the Rolls Royce category, four star fuel in the form of a first class diet containing no junk food, is recommended.

5   Go for walks in areas where children can run and explore in safety. Freedom to run and run, to shout and shout, is a rare treat today. Long grass to throw oneself into without reservation, only to jump up and repeat the performance, has to be experienced to be believed. This pleasure is simulated in rooms filled with foam cushions or coloured tunnels, over an inflated mattress. Nature provides the original, it just takes a little perserverance to find the right spot.

6   Teach children to sit quietly and wait for something to happen, especially in the countryside. Teach them to listen and to select meaningful sounds from those around them. Once it is understood how complex a skill this is to operate effectively, in most nursery or infant environments, it will be appreciated that the problems encountered are beyond many young children. Nevertheless in such situations one may often hear adults remonstrating with children for 'not listening'. How are they to know what they are supposed to select as meaningful, at any point in time? How are they to demonstrate such skill without regular guidance and practice. The nursery nurse is often in a position to stimulate the development of listening skills.

7   Use leaves for rubbings, pointing out obvious differences, and naming those with characteristic properties. Cut out the individual leaves after using seasonal colours to produce the rubbings, and mount in a large tree shape as a wall decoration.

Avoid asking the children to fill large shapes with crumpled balls of coloured tissue, unless the only objective, is that of social inter-action. There is little stimulation otherwise.

8   Press, or roll over with a rolling pin, a large well-shaped leaf onto a smooth, thin, flat piece of clay. Cut away surplus clay and gently curl the remaining shape into a realistic autumn leaf. Ideally this should be baked in a kiln, but some clays can simply dry out. If a Baker's clay is used it can be dried out in a normal gas or electric oven.

9   An easy recipe to follow to produce chocolate leaves involves melting some chocolate in a bowl over hot water. Remove the bowl from the heat and place on a low table so that the children can observe, and then participate. Take some rose leaves and gently draw them across the surface of the chocolate, the underside of the leaf being coated. Carefully place each leaf separately on a piece of foil and leave in a cool place or in the fridge for a short time. The leaves will come away from the chocolate leaving a beautiful replica which can be used for cake decoration or eaten.

PHYSICS

Physics for small children is their acquaintance with the properties of substances they will encounter in everyday life. Substances such as wood, metal, liquids and gases, and the relationships between these. Also the building up of experiences which lead towards an intelligent and logical prediction of what will happen next, given certain infor-mation. Think about the path which a cone shaped object will follow if set in motion. Think about a cylinder's movement, what is the difference and how do you think you know?

Through discovery, children will learn a great deal about their physical world, but a careful manipulation of the environment, can cause this learning to be of a richer nature. Provide items of wood, metal, plastic or any other suitable material for use in the water trough (Fig. 10.2). Some will float, others sink, but there is no need to constantly point this out. Listening to the children can often confirm, or otherwise, if concepts are established.

1 Provide magnets for the children to use in an unstructured way. Make a simple game by marking a winding road with perhaps a roundabout or pedestrian crossing on the board or card. Test that there is a strong magnet available which will attract through the board or card. The child has to guide a metal object representing a vehicle and take in on a journey keeping on the road and negotiating any obstacles.

2 If possible allow children to play with some of the executive toys which use magnets as their base. It may be possible to borrow these, as it is unlikely the toys would come to any harm.

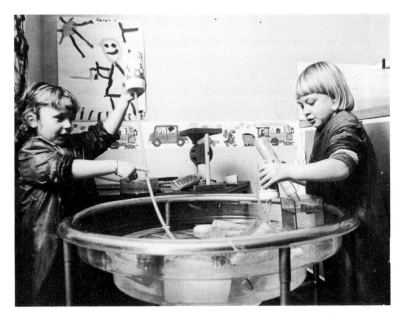

Fig. 10.2 A trough filled with water can provide first hand knowledge of basic physical properties.

3 Present problems to the children. Concentrate on movement: movement of a heavy object, playing on a see-saw with an adult, moving water from one level to another, using the scientific principles. Solutions to such problems can be worked towards in a practical way.

CHEMISTRY

Chemistry is the science which is concerned with the properties of substances, and their combinations and reactions.

1 There are plenty of opportunities to introduce principles associated with chemistry, when following the normal everyday routine. What happens when sugar is stirred into a cup of hot tea? It dissolves. Can you see it, where does it go, can it be reclaimed? What happens to water when it becomes very hot, or very cold? Make an ice hand by freezing a rubber glove full of water. Freeze a bottle of milk, what happens to the foil top? It rises on a cylindrical frozen milk lollipop. Some things melt, others dissolve, what is the difference?

2 Use some indoor fireworks as visual illustration for an appropriate story. The 'Porridge Pot' for example, which boiled over and could not be stopped. Make absolutely sure that the opportunity is taken to emphasize the necessity for taking safety precautions, whenever matches are used. Point out that this is a job for adults only, so that children may enjoy watching.

3 Take a large bottle or carboy, fill it with water and add a few drops of vegetable dye gently at the top. The patterns made by single or mixed colours are beautiful, and the children will be fascinated.

4 Make a 'witch's potion' by adding coloured inks to a large glass container of water.

5 One of the most satisfying ways of experiencing chemical reaction is to organize cooking sessions. These will be covered in a comprehensive way in the following section.

6 Make up a solution of liquid detergent and water, for bubble blowing. A little glycerine may make the bubbles longer lasting. The children will enjoy watching the bubbles float away, enjoy trying to catch the biggest ones, and will be fascinated by the colours trapped by the sunlight.

Similar colours may be found in puddles contaminated by petrol.

If these are in a safe position, the colours can be swirled with a stick. Discuss why plain water is not suitable for bubble blowing.

COOKERY

Cookery, with children both as active participants and observers (see Fig. 10.3), can encompass a wider variety of learning and formation of concepts than many adults realize. Reading recipes; recording, weighing, and measuring of ingredients; temperature control; use of electricity or gas; conduction of heat through metal; basic nutrition; chemical reactions; origin of ingredients; timing; cultural patterns of recipe; and ways of eating are only some of the areas which are covered, often without even realizing it. Added to all this is the social occasion of eating in a group with friends, relatives, family, even strangers.

Having appreciated the value of cookery it is necessary to explore situations in which the children can gain maximum benefit without

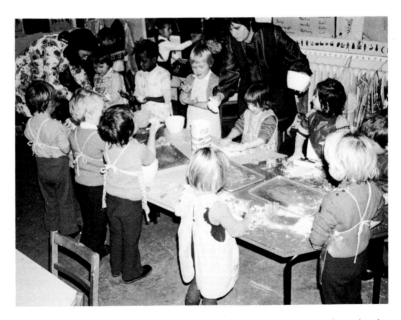

Fig. 10.3 It is difficult to think of a skill which is not expressed or developed through the group activity of cooking.

contrivance. If you intend to plan a session during which the children can participate, remember to keep the group small, well-supervised, and adequately provided with ingredients and utensils. Make sure that the dish can be divided easily into pieces or portions, which can be shared for taking home, or eaten together at school or nursery. Buns in bun cases, flapjacks, cornflake crunchies, rock buns, peppermint creams, jam tarts, and biscuits are recommended. If you are good at making a running commentary, a demonstration of a more complicated dish can be entertaining and informative for the children. Tasting afterwards is a necessary part of the whole proceedings.

All learning takes place through the senses, and a combination usually establishes any learning in a more effective way. Cookery stimulates: listening, and therefore *hearing*, by the need to follow instructions; *seeing*, by observing stages in a process, or identifying ingredients; *smelling*, by enjoying the food before, during, and after cooking; *touching*, by handling while preparing ingredients; and *tasting*, before, during, and after preparation.

Please note that sometimes the value of some experiences will override the need for overzealous attention to hygiene. Reluctant eaters or those recovering from illness can often help to plan and prepare their own meals. It is much more likely that they will feel like sampling the results of their own labours. Do not worry if children prefer some foods raw, in unusual combinations or order. Ask yourself 'Why not?' and see how difficult it is to present a logical argument.

Many families rarely sit down together for a meal. Work, television, and a tendency to drift away from a traditional family lifestyle especially in adolescence, has contributed towards this situation. Consequently, some young mothers simply never set a table in an attractive way, and present a family meal as a social occasion. Teach the children how to do this properly at lunch time, by having a set of cutlery, china, condiments, place mats or table-cloth, napkins/serviettes, flowers, even candles, and supervise the laying of the table. Let small groups take it in turns and encourage, even insist upon, 'special behaviour'.

On festive occasions or other specific days, support the tradition of eating special foods: on Shrove Tuesday make pancakes, at Easter boil and decorate eggs. Nests can be made of shedded wheat, mixed into melted chocolate, and formed into shapes, then filled with sugar eggs. On Hallowe'en toffee apples can be prepared, on bonfire night, toffee and baked potatoes, and at Christmas, mince pies can be made. In many areas there are children from a variety of cultural backgrounds whose festivals and celebrations can be shared within the school or nursery environment. An exchange of such ideas is an excellent way of building relationships.

ART

Art is more than brushes, paints and paper. It is the expression of an individual in two or three dimensional form. The aim should be towards the provision of the widest range of materials as possible. All sorts of writing and drawing materials, and different types of surfaces present a variety of experiences and outcome. Dry powder paint, for instance, dropped onto wet paper causes a very different product to emerge, compared with the more familiar wet paint and dry paper.

There are numerous publications written around the theme of art and young children (see p. 193). A few ideas will be offered here, but this will serve only to scratch the surface of those which can be used.

1   Take a wall-paper sample book, and select those pages on which the designs are in strong relief, or embossed. These can be cut by the adult or the children, or both, into various shapes. These shapes may be geometric, or part of a collage picture, and should be mounted on stiff card possibly from good supermarket boxes. By placing paper over the finished construction, fixed with paper clips or tape, rubbings can be taken using wax crayons. These are very satisfying for the children to do, there is no possibility of failure, and the potential range of standard and complexity is almost infinite.

2   Printing is a popular activity with young children, especially if they first make their own blocks. These can easily be made from off-cuts of wood of almost any shape, as long as these can be grasped easily. Cut potatoes can also be used for printing. Hand printing never fails to be successful (Fig. 10.4). Awkward shapes can have a large 'head' glued on the top for easier handling.

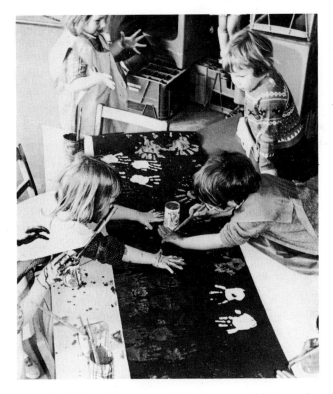

Fig. 10.4 Hand printing gives personal involvement which together with the immediate result are ingredients for success.

Random patterns can be formed from string simply curled onto the block, which is covered in glue. Representive patterns take a little more time and care.

Felt, thin rubber, plastic tiles, linoleum, cork, polystyrene all provide suitable material for making patterns for block printing. Some of these may not last very long, but their value is reflected in the creativity expressed by the children, and the freedom exercised in their decision-making.

Do not use ready made tools if at all possible, making them with the children can be a legitimate learning experience. Never use such an activity simply to fill time.

3 Ask the children to cover completely a piece of paper with bright colours from waxed crayons. Hide this under a coating of indian ink, which should then be allowed to dry completely. Demonstrate how, by scratching at the surface gently, the colours will emerge in any desired pattern or picture. Once again there is complete freedom of interpretation, and an element of surprise, together with ensured success.

This last criterion is vital. Any artistic work is a disclosure of part of the soul of the artist. The piece becomes an extension of the artist and renders the artist vulnerable. It is so easy to damage the confidence and self image of the children by insensitively discussing their works. By ensuring success, some methods of presentation serve to strengthen and improve self image, therefore they are particularly appropriate for the withdrawn or nervous child.

4 Bubble painting is always successful too, and very effective on display. Powder paint is made up with water into a consistency which can be 'blown' into bubbles through a straw. Various colours are put separately into containers with different shaped and sized tops. Bubbles are blown, so that they rise above the level of the top, then a piece of paper is laid gently over. As the bubbles burst a pattern is left on the paper. After some experimentation colour combinations can become quite sophisticated.

5 Marbling inks are available through art suppliers with instructions for use.

CRAFTS

Crafts will be looked at in relation to making things, although it is not easy to distinguish between art and craft even for the academic exercise of presentation. To avoid confusion let it be accepted here that in all art there is craft and vice versa.

The activities which are most familiar in the world of young children are those of modelling with clay or junk, and working with wood.

1 Modelling with clay relates closely to modelling with plasticine or Playdo, but each has particular properties, and children should have the opportunity to practise with each. They learn to appreciate the particular character of different materials, and that certain 'rules' are attributable to them. They find that cold plasticine is not easily malleable, but that as it warms it becomes more responsive. They discover that clay needs to be stored in a certain environment to be suitable for modelling at all. They also find that when they have spent much time, effort and thought on making their model, some kindly adult nearly always asks them to 'roll it up into a nice ball again'. Strangely enough this ritual is usually followed without much comment, but it does not reflect the importance placed on creativity and expression, even accepting the cost of clay, and plasticine.

Provide 'tools' which will make patterns in the clay and try 'rolling' over a piece of net, or string vest to produce quick interesting textures. Through basic materials such as clay, the whole range of skill may be observed. This will commence with exploration and experimentation, lead on to practice towards refinement, and result in illustrations of creativity. This developmental path may be traced through the acquisition of other skills, such as cooking, gymnastics, knitting, woodwork, mechanics, even language. There is a wide range, but all may serve as illustrative models for the processes observed towards true creativity, reflected in many unique achievements.

2 Creativity may be found in any situation, where children have been provided with a large selection of junk materials together with suitable fixatives to join them to each other (Fig. 10.5). If different surfaces will need to be joined, then different glues will need to be available and paints must be checked to be sure they will cover the surfaces to be used. Nothing is more disappointing for a child than to see his or her model fall apart as it is carried proudly across the room to show his or her mother.

During the time allowed for the construction of models, try to give each child a period of peace, during which time he or she can think and plan. When it seems appropriate listen to the language and join in, do not dominate.

It is not difficult to appreciate the value of such sessions. The children make decisions, plan ahead, select materials, look at size and proportion, decide on colour and always achieve an end result, which to them is usually satisfactory. If this is not so, they can often benefit from self appraisal. More materials can be provided so a fresh attempt may be made to achieve success.

3 Wood should be available in its various forms: solid, shavings,

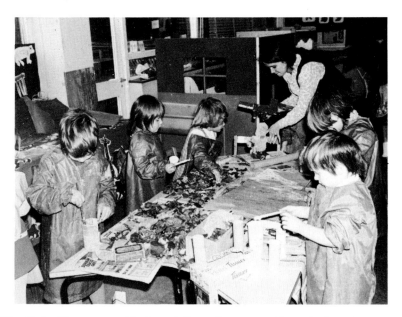

Fig. 10.5   The success of junk modelling relies on as wide a selection of materials as possible being available. *Note* only empty boxes of matches should be given to the children to build from.

and sawdust. If possible, let the children see how each is formed, by visiting a workshop, or demonstrating yourself. Always provide tools which will efficiently perform the job for which they are designed. 'Toy' tools are not satisfactory, as they are usually too light. But small proper hammers, planes and screwdrivers are quite safe if sensibly supervised. One must be prepared for an occasional lack of judgement, and there will be a sore finger or thumb now and again. It is impossible to totally prevent children from hurting themselves, and at the same time, enable them to follow a rich programme of experiences. Much better to educate them to be aware of dangers, to anticipate intelligently, and to develop a responsibility for self. With balsa wood and glue, off-cuts and nails, rough pieces of wood and a carving tool, many figments of imagination are nursed and beaten into reality.

A forerunner to woodcarving can be provided by working with soap or block salt, but this is expensive. Shavings can be used, either for part of, or the whole of, a collage picture, causing an effective three-dimensional feature. Finished work may be sprayed with coloured paint or, gold or silver paint. This must be done outside, in a sheltered place, as many authorities are conscious of the potential danger of using such aerosol canisters in a confined environment.

Shavings, very carefully handled will form excellent shapes for mobiles, especially if hung in the path of air movement. Sawdust can be used for shaking over glued areas of a painting or design, or as a material for use in containers instead of sand. Naturally it will not hold its shape like damp sand, but even this difference adds to a child's experience and knowledge of his or her world. Sawdust is also useful for demonstrating the relationship of mass to weight.

Have a large block of wood firmly anchored in some way, and allow the children to practise hitting nails into it, aiming to keep them straight. This is quite a complex skill, and many adults find it difficult to perform.

Many other materials can be used for making things: fabric, paper, card, knitting wool, paper maché, to name but a few. There is always a pleasure and pride in achieving a finished result, and it is up to the adult to encourage, even insist upon, a high standard of workmanship. Children know, and have little respect for, the tolerance of the misguided adult who, in a patronizing fashion, accepts, and even praises, work which has taken little effort, time, or thought.

USEFUL REFERENCES

The books named here are suggested as suitable texts on crafts which will provide and stimulate new ideas.

Make Your Own Musical Instruments. M. Mandell & R. E. Wood. New York, Sterling Publishing Company (1982).

Starting With Papier Mâché. C. J. Alkema. Little Craft Book Series. New York, Sterling Publishing Company (1974).

Greetings Cards You Can Make. C. J. Alkema. Little Craft Book Series. New York, Sterling Publishing Company (1975).

The Zoo. Needlecraft for young children. B. Snook. London, B T Batsford (1975).

Fun With Felt. V. Janitch. London, Kaye and Ward in association with Australia, Methuen and New Zealand, Hicks Smith (1978).

Paper Folding and Modelling. A. Van Breda. London, Faber and Faber (1964).

Kites. M. McPhum. Illustrated by E. Carr. London, Macdonald Education (1979).

Making a Miniature Village. G. R. Williams. London, Faber and Faber (1970).

More Masks and Party Hats. R. Brown. Aylesbury, Bucks, Goodchild (John) Publishers (1983).

Third Book of Wooden Toys. W. G. Alton. London, Mills & Boon (1974).

More Things to Make. Devised and drawn by R. Brown. Aylesbury, Bucks, Goodchild (John) Publishers in conjunction with the Girl Guide Association (1977).

Make Things Grandma Made. M. Stapleton. London, Studio Vista (1975).

Doll Making. A. V. Dean. Illustrated by M. Mills. East Sussex, Wayland Publishers (1974).

Paper Cutting. F. Temko. Illustrated by S. Madison. Tadworth, Surrey, World's Work (1974).

Crafts and Toys From Around the World. A. J. Newsome. Tadworth, Surrey, World's Work (1972).

Fun With Picture Projects. T. Hart. London, Kaye and Ward (1973).

Fun With Shapes and Patterns. G. C. Payne, London, Kaye and Ward (1974).

Chapter 11
Stories and Games

TELLING STORIES

The telling of stories knows no boundaries, either of time or culture. Certain people are better than others at demonstrating this skill, and in some societies there will be a regular teller of stories, often an elder member of the community. The stories he or she will tell are usually based upon personal early experiences, or are the traditional lore passed from generation to generation within a specific cultural framework.

Children never tire of hearing about when they were babies, adults of talking about their childhood, and old people find great pleasure in reminiscing. The older they are, the more fascinating are the stories they tell.

It follows that stories are not necessarily based upon fiction, some of the best and most fantastic are based on fact, and real life experiences. Also, although books have an essential part to play, they should never be regarded as the essential equipment for the story teller. Thinking carefully about it, the most pleasurable story experience is often told directly person to person. The contact made through body language, facial expression, and eye to eye contact, creates a special quality of communication.

Just as with a good joke teller, some people are naturally good story tellers. Those who find it difficult to master and enjoy this skill need to appreciate its importance, and then practise, following a few tips, until they enjoy the activity as much as is possible. Children are a most receptive audience, and will offer the nervous newcomer to story telling, every encouragement to repeat the performance. Each child is offered a similar experience, yet each interprets it in an individual way (Fig. 11.1).

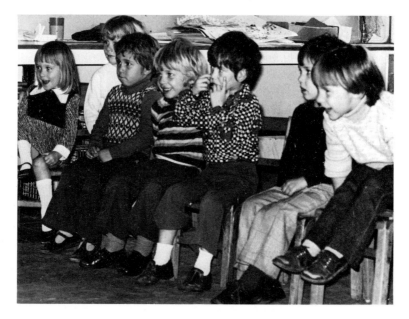

Fig. 11.1   A variety of responses to the same story illustrates the individuality of each child.

Setting the scene

What useful purpose is served by story telling? Firstly there is the human contact, physical if possible, certainly social, emotional and often intellectual. Physically there should be a minimum distance between teller and receiver. If one or two children are involved, then sitting on a knee or in a large chair enfolded by an arm creates an ideal situation. If a small group is involved, then the listeners should be almost on the same level as the teller. It is common to see a group of small children tipping their heads back to look at the individual, either talking to them or telling a story. This is a most uncomfortable position to hold for any length of time, and illustrates the inability of many adults to truly place themselves in 'other people's shoes'. So, comfort is the first criterion to consider for all parties concerned. This includes warmth, freedom from hunger or thirst, or a need to visit the lavatory. All these will affect concentration and enjoyment, the latter will dominate all other thoughts. These may all sound simple, but a successful session does rely on the minimum of distractions and the most positive environment. Often failure is felt personally when it is really due to inadequate preparation. So, secondly preparation deserves some closer attention.

The time of each session of uninterrupted story should be roughly two and half times the average age of the group. The result of this calculation will give a number which equals the minutes suggested. For example, a group of 3-year-olds will listen well and be able to concentrate for about 7-8 minutes. After this period, a different activity or an extension to the original one will be happily entered into.

Children will need an opportunity to move around and to talk, so an extension could be, one of playing different characters from the story. These activities need as much, if not more preparation than the story itself. This should be read through, timed, scanned for new words or concepts which can cause interruptions, and sifted for inappropiate content. Hansel and Gretel may not be suitable if a child has recently suffered a family breakdown. A child about to enter hospital, on the other hand, may benefit considerably through hearing one of the excellent informative stories written around this theme.

Thirdly, and linked to preparation, is to select the method to be used. There are many ways of telling a story, some of them use a book to a greater or lesser degree.

Methods of story telling

FLANNELGRAPH

It is easy and cheap to make a flannelgraph out of stiff card or light wood covered with felt-like material. The furry side of lint works well, as do the soft fluffy man-made fabrics. A dark colour will not become grubby too quickly, but care must be taken to contrast the fabrics used for mounting shapes, in order that they show up clearly. The colours do not necessarily need to be accurately representative, all sorts of scraps and oddments will present original ideas.

The flannelgraph can be built up as the tale progresses, and often this can be done by the children. The beauty of the system is that participation is real, and the picture which emerges is always different. If time and patience are available, small flannelgraphs can be made so that the children can build their own pictures. Obviously this allows for more than one extra and purposeful activity, preparing the chosen shapes for mounting, skills such as cutting, matching and proportional representation will be practised and evaluated.

PUPPETS

As with a flannelgraph the children can be involved in making puppets using characters from favourite stories. Once the adult has demonstrated what fun it can be to give these toys a character, and control their speed and actions, other play situations will develop. Using puppets helps the more withdrawn child to participate actively, as he or she need not necessarily appear, being behind a screen or curtain. In fact, even if not hidden from view, he or she feels more confident believing that attention is directed away from him or her, which is absolutely true. A 'stage' can be made out of very large cardboard boxes, a curtain and two chairs, or a table with a 'skirt' round it.

There are many sorts of puppets from the simple stick person made out of a paper plate and rod, through finger and glove puppets, to string puppets, of a complicated nature with many individual controls. They can be made from odds and ends, and thus are cheap to construct, and a large number can provide a good resource for stimulating story sessions.

TELEVISION BOX

A strong cardboard box can be used to make a television box. The best are those used to hold bottles of wine, or any other similar commodity. A 'window' is cut from one side, as neatly as possible. It is essential to make such equipment using the best tools and materials available, and taking great care to work as cleanly as possible. The highest standards should always be set when performing the simplest tasks. As Bill Shankly once said 'When I was in the army, if I had a job to do, even if it was cleaning a floor, I'd try to make sure that my floor was better than anyone else's.' If everyone had a similar approach to each job there would not be much wrong with the world.

Adults should always demonstrate through their own performance that a philosophy such as Bill Shankly's is worth adopting. Therefore, when working with small children always encourage them towards a good job, rather than a satisfactory one. When making equipment for or with them, insist on high standard.

The carefully cut box can be decorated by the children, then they can each depict a part of a familiar story on a piece of paper cut to fit the screen. These pictures are attached to rods suspended in logical order inside the box, and removed at the appropriate moment in the story, to present the next 'scene'.

DRAMATIC PLAY

Children involve themselves quite regularly in spontaneous dramatic play. This can be observed in most home corners, playgrounds, and any place where children gather to play. It is usually unplanned and undirected, and possesses a special quality due to this absence of adult intervention. It is legitimate to tap this skill and use it to interpret a story. Either some children can present the drama, and others act as the audience, or the whole group can enjoy the experience of projecting themselves as a joint activity. For example, take *The Selfish Giant* by Oscar Wilde. All the children can be the angry giant, the children sad, and then the children happy. They could be the trees, blossoming into life, through the change in the giant's heart. Most stories will offer some possibilities, but it is worth having a few which present a particularly rich fund of ideas for transforming into a dramatic experience. Once more, an extension may be the preparation of dressing up clothes, or even scenery.

SEQUENCE STORIES

All participants are used in an active way in the telling of sequence stories. One person starts the story, and then on an agreed signal the next person, or some other chosen at random, continues the sequence. A tactful leader will notice when an individual has reached a natural turning point or has dried up, and will signal a change. Added to progressive rotation there are methods such as spinning a pointer, throwing a dice, or throwing a bean bag or similar article to the chosen person. This will avoid the participants preparing their piece rather than listening to the other contributors.

WORD LUCKY DIP

The group select some key words, put them in a hat, and a certain number are drawn out. These words must then be used to tell a story. The stories may be very short, and a few individuals can be offered the opportunity to demonstrate the funniest way in which they can use all the words in a short story. This is obviously a way in which word recognition can be practised in an amusing fashion.

RAG BAG

The stories told from the rag bag can be made very personal to the group of children, and if appropriate to any child or children within it. The only prop needed is a bag full of fabric scraps containing as much variety as possible. Bits of leather, oilcloth, or string can be included. The idea is to search around in the bag, preferably blind-folded or ask a child to do the same. One piece will be selected and then the story teller will weave a story around the imaginary life of that piece of fabric or material. It is a good ploy to include the children in the tale as much as possible. They love it, and for obvious reasons become very involved, and therefore practise the skill of concentration in an attractive way. For example, on 'finding' a piece of furry fabric (acquired from Michael's mother with some information):

'Once upon a time, I was part of a big heavy roll of fabric just like this delivered to a large store in Croydon (all such details will be adapted). One morning, just after Bonfire Night, a very nice lady came into the store and found her way to the department where patterns and fabrics are sold. She was already thinking about Christmas, and had decided to make a dressing gown for her little boy Michael.

Michael had been particularly good lately (for some reason) and his Mother wanted to do something special for him to show once again how much she loved him. I knew that I would be able to keep him warm and cosy on chilly winter evenings and I did so hope that she would choose me. . . .

The story can be told in the first or third person. The former is fun to use especially when the cloth is experiencing being made up and tickled by the pins and needles. Anyone with a fertile mind can make up the most interesting and exciting stories, using this idea as a starting point. An extension may be, asking the children to bring a scrap from home in order to tell their own story.

The scraps can be mounted onto a collage, building up to form a unique history of the stories told over a period of time. The children will probably find favourites. These can be told again and again, the beauty being that each time they will change a little, as folk lore does when passed from person to person unrecorded.

MUSIC STORIES

Although the word opera is a familiar one the experience of such, is not common to most children. It is the adult 'music story' and demands a special type of appreciation and understanding.

All children will enjoy, and actively participate in stories told with musical accompaniment. This can range from simple percussion used to represent giants' footsteps to extracts from light classical music used at intervals to illustrate mood or action. The children may listen or move appropriately to the music, a combination of each seems a perfect recipe.

One of the most familiar 'music stories' is that of *Peter and the Wolf*, but with a bit of time spent planning and recording, many others lend themselves to this method. Most of the children will watch some television and will quickly identify music used to indicate suspense, tranquillity, or happiness. As they get older, they will be able to say 'It's going to be all right; listen to the music.' Music can be integrated into almost any of the suggested methods of story telling and should never be considered in isolation.

CHORUS STORIES

Stories with short repetitive sections occuring at regular intervals are always well received. Once again it is the pleasure of involvement which is appealing. Think of the positive participation at Pantomimes when the community chorus is displayed for the audience and everyone can join in. Coming into this category are the 'Gingerbread Man', 'The Three Bears', and 'Billy Goats Gruff'. All these have a fear element, but in spite of that, are usually well requested and would probably figure in a 'Top Twenty' list of popular stories for the under 8's, especially when used as a group experience.

CUMULATIVE STORIES

These are stories which offer similar values to the 'Chorus' type. There is sufficient repetition on a building basis to allow for real participation 'Chicken Licken', 'The Enormous Turnip' and 'We're Going on a Bear Hunt' come into this category. The 'Bear Hunt' is very popular, having actions and funny sounds, as well as the more usual word form.

RHYMES

Most of those who work with young children will manage to acquire a good repertoire of finger and action rhymes. It is a good idea to make some personal recordings of these, to be used as a trigger during sessions. It is surprising how elusive some of them become, when faced with the situation of many pairs of expectant waiting eyes. They are useful for one's own children and are invaluable if returning to work after a gap of some years.

There are many books of rhymes available (see p. 208). Nursery rhymes tend to repeat what the parent has used, and are of limited value, so ideally a selection of the familiar, together with the new, is ideal. It is a pity that young children tend to be deprived of the quality of rhyme and verse which may lead to a love of poetry. There is a tendency later on in schools to present poetry in such a fashion, that young people avoid it altogether on a permanent basis, or at least for many years. It follows that those entering vocational courses, have little or no ready source material on which to draw. Part of the culture of any society lies in its literature and there are many beautiful poems written especially for children. There is no other way, but for those who really care about such things, to learn a selection of poems, and share them with the very young, who have no way of knowing of such treasures, unless someone makes the effort to enable these experiences to be available.

Poems can be used as source material for other activities, and then more can be searched for once they have served their purpose. This experience can help to lay the foundations for future skills and imaginative use of language.

BOOKS

It would be untrue to say that without books we would not have stories. Stories came before the book and books should be used as an invaluable source, not an essential crutch. Children need to familiarize themselves with books in order to master the skill of reading, and share experiences beyond their own, enabling them to make decisions later in life about the information and literature they wish to have access to.

It is now considered less important simply to provide many books and more important to share a few with the child, introducing the habits of left to right progression and linking the printed word with spoken language. Books, ideally, can become friends, informing, comforting, emotionally moving, even frightening their readers, but invariably broadening their horizons and enriching their intellectual capacity.

It is relevant to suggest here that any person working with children should collect some books. To start with, a selection of traditional stories, some familiar, some new, of varying lengths, together with a comprehensive collection of poems, rhymes and jingles, would be sufficient. To this add the personal book of rhymes already suggested. It is difficult to recommend type and quantity of illustrations as this is very much a matter of taste, as is the quality of script. A good guide is that the more expensive a book, on the whole, the better it will be regarding quality of content and illustration.

If visiting school bazaars, or local charity fairs, it is possible to find second hand books at a very reasonable price. The annuals are not recommended as good material for stories or poetry, but may provide good pictures for cutting out or for making work cards. The stiff backs should be saved, as card is very expensive and frequently desirable for making teaching or learning aids. Libraries sell books which have quite a bit of life left in them, and are very reasonably priced.

Confidence will be gained very quickly through a few successful and happy story sessions, and such sessions will then be anticipated joyfully by both the teller and the told. It is worth preparing well and taking great care not to cut short this activity.

In the chapter on planning group activities, it will be easy to appreciate how a successful story or poetry session can be the starting point for many more valuable learning opportunities. The end of a story may be the beginning of something else.

GAMES

The games looked at in this section will be those which contain either formal patterning, or some rules. The spontaneous games which develop in a random fashion, i.e. role play, are discussed in Chapter 10.

For these games, it is a question of having to know how to play, or being ready to learn how to play, e.g. during very early hide and seek, a baby will find a hidden object under a blanket, and then wait patiently for it to be hidden again. Already there is the understanding of taking a specific part in a social ritual. From this simple activity, a development can be traced through party games of 'Hunt the Thimble' and 'Sardines' to the fairly sophisticated 'Treasure Hunt' and a related sport, that of orienteering. This is a complex system of finding points on a map, where machines stamp a card, proving that certain locations have been visited. It is another illustration of the fascination of 'Hide and Seek'.

Ring games, i.e. 'Ring O Roses', 'Farmers in the Dell', 'Poor Mary Sits a Weeping' and 'In and Out the Dusty Bluebells', offer participation for a flexibly sized group.

The words for these games are simple and the tunes easy for the amateur to learn. If any games are new, it is likely that they may be found on record or on tape. Failing this, experienced teachers or nursery nurses would probably be happy to make a recording with their own groups of children. This would be used as support during the time when a new game is being practised.

The repertoire offered by most individuals is relatively restricted, and many games that were popular a generation ago have virtually ceased to be played. Those who are working or plan to work with young children need to make the effort to acquire a good reportoire of games. Here are a few suggestions accompanied by the justification for their inclusion in the lives of children:

Ring O Roses
Farmers in the Dell
Poor Mary Sits a Weeping
Cobbler, Cobbler Mend my Shoe
Lucy Locket Lost her Pocket
In and Out the Dusty Bluebells
In and Out the Windows
The Big Ship Goes Through the Ally, Ally O
Hide and Seek
Skipping
Oranges and Lemons
Nuts in May
Froggie, Froggie May We Cross Your Water
Spin the Trencher
Hopscotch
Simon Says, or O'Grady Says
Hokey Cokey

This is a representative selection, and ideally the aim should be to be skilled enough to offer about ten such games. This means learning them sufficiently so there is a positive model for the children to follow. It is of little use to know part of the words or activities, better not to introduce any games with such inadequate preparation.

Experiencing the sort of games suggested, develops being socially orientated. The children learn to cooperate with each other, take turns, accept being out of the limelight, being disappointed, waiting for others to make decisions and taking part for the sake of the group, when at times they may prefer not to. There is no harm in persuading, or even insisting at times that everyone joins in. There are many occasions in life, when unpleasant tasks must be carried through, when for the sake of others, joining in is necessary. Strangely enough very often when the effort is made reluctantly, the resulting pleasure is surprisingly rewarding.

Board games

In most toy cupboards there will be a selection of board games. Many of these will have been acquired over a period of years and at traditional times for buying games. Most will not be played at all, some fairly frequently, and a small number will be so popular that they may even wear out and require replacement. The 'evergreens' are 'Monopoly' 'Snakes and Ladders', 'Ludo', 'Chess', 'Draughts', 'Cluedo', 'Scrabble', and many more. Some rely on chance, together with some decision-making as in Ludo and Snakes and Ladders. Others such as Monopoly require more decision-making, and Chess depends entirely on this and other skills of analysis. Similar skills are most useful throughout life.

Chess is a game suitable for all age groups, from 4 years old, for as long as mental facilities remain. It is a pity that more children are not introduced to it at an early age, as it is a stimulating way to develop the skills already mentioned. It also develops concentration, and the ability to think ahead through possible moves, in other words, to hypothesize and plan a strategy. All these skills are capable of becoming highly complex and it is usually the adult who decides that the young shall not be exposed to these experiences. This is unfortunate as it may lay good foundations for the development of higher intellectual functioning. It is suggested that all preschool children should have the opportunity to learn to play chess.

Card games

A pack of playing cards will probably present the widest range of games to the widest range of age groups.

Very young children can play matching games, identify shapes and recognize numbers, even using incomplete sets of cards. Selecting pairs and placing them at random, face down on a flat surface, is all that is needed to play 'Pelmanism'. The person who selects either by luck, observation and memory, or a combination of these, a matching pair, is allowed to score a point. The skills mentioned are developed together with 'waiting for a turn' and 'keeping to rules'. There are other games suitable for young children using a basic pack of cards. Amongst them are 'Snap', 'Beg O' my Neighbour', 'Families' (collecting four of a number) and 'Patience'.

The most complex game is probably that of 'Bridge'. This requires constant concentration, planning, anticipation and communication skills. It also demands a specific ability to remember the cards which have been played and by whom. It would seem out of place to find young children playing bridge in an infant school, and yet the game demands skills which would be beneficial to those children, when transferred to other intellectual and practical areas.

'Pontoon' if played for tokens will provide a useful vehicle for quick mathematical calculations. Risk-taking and decision-making are life skills experienced in safe and simple form in many card and board games. It is a pity that the terms 'playing games' should be often attributed to those activities of little educational value. The playing of games for some relates very closely to working life for others. For example the footballer, book illustrator, dancer, or disc jockey, earns a living, doing what may be referred to in another environment as 'playing'. Football, drawing, dancing, and chatting whilst listening to popular music, would hardly ever achieve high status in a normal school curriculum. Nevertheless the supporting skills required to follow any of these activities seriously, are based in the more familiar reading, writing and arithmetic. Young children could certainly acquire many, if not most, of the skills of life through the vehicles of game playing.

SUMMARY

This section aims to persuade the reader to revaluate an area which should receive more attention, in the planning of activities for young children. It is necessary to appreciate that by using games a wide variety of desirable skills may be developed.

USEFUL REFERENCES

The books named here are suggested as suitable sources for poems and rhymes. There is certainly a fund of varied material with something to suit everyone.

A Child's Garden Verse. R. L. Stevenson. Illustrated by Brian Wildsmith. Oxford, Oxford University Press (1966).

Oh, Such Foolishness. Poems selected by W. Cole. Pictures by T. de Paola. London, Methuen (1978).

A Thread of Gold. An anthology of poetry for the very young. Compiled by E. Graham. Illustrated by M. Gill. London, The Bodley Head (1964).

Days Are Where We Live, and Other Poems. Compiled by J. Bennett. Illustrated by M. Roffey. London, The Bodley Head (1981).

Hist Whist. Poems of magic and mystery, witches and ghosts. Collected by D. Saunders. Illustrated by K. Wyatt. London, Evans Brothers Ltd (1975).

The Batsford Book of Light Verse for Children. Edited by G. Ewart. Illustrated by N. Bentley. London, B T Batsford Ltd (1978).

Nursery Songs and Carols, with Music. F. Waters. London, Westerham Press (1971).

Stuff and Nonsense. Compiled by M. Dagan. Illustrated by Deborah Niland. Glasgow, Collins (1974).

The Swinging Rainbow. Poems for the young. Selected by H. Sergeant. Illustrated by B. Denyer. London, Evans Brothers Ltd (1979).

If You Should Meet a Crocodile, and Other Verse. Compiled by M. Mayo. Illustrated by C. Barker. London, Kaye and Ward (1974).

Fives, Sixes and Sevens. A collection of poetry for the very young. Compiled by M. Stephenson. Illustrated by D. Wrigley. London, Frederick Warne (Publishers) (1968).

Chapter 12
Observing Children

It is essential to develop the skills of observation. This skill is not only useful, but also a vital component within the overall assessment of a child. It may be the vehicle through which warning signals indicating the onset of illness, handicap or child abuse, can be diagnosed through professional interpretation of accurately recorded facts.

To develop sensitive skills of precise observation, student nursery nurses will practise making records throughout their period of training and education. This 2 year period prepares the students to be competent as junior members within team situations. They will, on their first appointments, learn to transfer the basic skills acquired to more specialized situations.

It is easily forgotten by newly qualified nursery nurses and their supervisors that they are on the threshold of new learning opportunities. They have not completed their education nor, hopefully, will they ever cease to be receptive to new information and knowledge and the opportunity to acquire skills. Learning continues throughout life, no-one ever reaches the stage at which the process can be called complete. Not only is learning necessary for life itself but it has been proved that people remain active and healthier in other respects, when learning activities take place during the later stages of life.

THE FUNCTION OF OBSERVATION

According to the National Nursery Examination Board (NNEB) December 1981, the function of observation is 'To promote the integration of theoretical knowledge and understanding of children's growth with practice so that through the precise identification of what children are doing now, an effective contribution can be made to meet their present and further needs.'

209

As students become increasingly familiar with normal patterns of development and expected stages at relative chronological ages, they will begin to identify areas of possible concern. It almost becomes 'second nature' for the experienced observer to be alerted to such areas before even embarking upon the exercise of detailed observation records. Such records are necessary to present evidence to the appropriate professional that the concern is supported by concrete facts.

METHODS OF RECORDING

Practitioners may develop preferred methods of recording, professionals may request that a certain pattern be presented. It is, therefore, important that the student has the opportunity to practise various methods. Some of the most common are:
1 Time sampling,
2 Event sampling,
3 Using prepared schedules,
4 Illustrating stages of an identified developmental process, e.g. dressing,
5 Verbatim recording of a dialogue or small group conversation,
6 Target child,
7 Comparative observations.

CRITERIA

Throughout the range certain criteria should be adhered to.

Permission is usually required from someone, the parent if the observation is to be made at home or, if in the practical placement, the appropriate teacher, nursery nurse or other responsible person. It is common practice to avoid using the child's real name in order to ensure confidentiality. Students' notes have been left on trains or buses, or simply carelessly put down in the nursery or school.

Information such as age, sex, size of family and general background are usually simple to acquire. Other useful and possibly important items may be gathered without deliberate inquisition. Listening is auditory observation, and conversations between children themselves and between child and parent can be helpful. It may be difficult if confidences are passed but if such items lead to a better understanding of the child they may justifiably be recorded for the exercise without using names. It may at such times be advisable to ask a senior member of staff, whether what has been recorded is significant. Even when there is no plan to make a specific observation, it is a good idea to develop the habit of carrying around a small note book and pencil. Some of the most interesting events take place unexpectedly. Just as newspaper photographers carry their cameras as a constant tool, pencil and paper should be to student nursery nurses.

Avoid making personal remarks and offering opinions within the script of an observation. It should aim towards a true reflection or objective record of what was actually seen or heard or both. Aim also to use groups of young children as well as the individuals more commonly represented, to build up a file of mixed observations. This file should at the end of the 2 year course, contain a minimum of 50 observations covering the following range of study areas (NNEB 1981):

a Physical growth and development.
b Development of communication skills.
c Development of cognitive skills.
d Variety of emotional expression and behaviour revealed in different experiences.
e Social development and relationships.
f Specific activities related to creative arts, growing independence, daily living.
g Wider learning capabilities including 5- to 7-year-old gifted children.
h Developmental patterns (preferably through the longitudinal observation of an individual child).
i Children with special needs.

Time sampling

Making a decision about how long a period to observe, between what intervals these observations should be made and for how long the serial should last are involved in time sampling.

TOTAL ACTIVITIES

A child may be observed for a couple of minutes at 20 minute intervals, for five consecutive mornings or afternoons. This exercise will provide a good illustration of the overall pattern of activity. It avoids a typical behaviour being accepted as representative, and if such a method is followed at intervals of 2-3 months an informative picture of progress will be illustrated.

At times when the child's or children's behaviour is especially exciting or interesting there is a strong temptation to continue the recording beyond the predetermined time span. To do this is to negate the object of the exercise and the resulting document will not be truly balanced and, therefore, cannot be accurately interpreted. Apply self discipline and stick to the plans made.

SPECIFIC ASPECTS

Together with the time sampling of total activities observed, another method is to focus on a specific aspect of behaviour. This must, once again, be decided in advance and the decision adhered to. If a child, for instance, seems to be more aggressive, withdrawn, immobile, dominant, lacking in initiative or negative, a series of samples may support such an impression or vice versa. The temptation to record other incidents must be overcome, some sample periods may record nothing. This, however, is a vital component which contributes towards the whole real 'picture'. This method of observation may also serve to illustrate that general impressions are not always accurate.

The tutor will need to be precise about definition of terms. What one individual will perceive as aggression, for instance, may well appear to another as 'strong leadership'. It can be useful for more than one student to observe the same situation, working from similar sets of instructions and definitions of terms. It is almost certain that the results will vary.

Event sampling

Specific events are either predetermined, the student being directed to wait for a particularly interesting incident, or a routine activity may be used as the focus. The guide could be:

1 Observe and record in as much detail as possible a child between 2 years old and 2½ years old (5-5½ years) playing with building blocks or bricks alone or within a small group.

2 When there is conflict between two children of any age, observe and record what happens. If possible say what led up to the incident and how and if it is resolved.

3 Observe a child who is learning to achieve independence in dressing or feeding.

With adaptation these exercises could be carried out in any basic training situation. Specialized ones relating to children with individual needs or comparative analyses, for example, can be fitted into the 2 year programme if details are available early enough. The student can then make such observations when the occasion arises. Some students may also welcome the idea of free choice for a number of assignments.

These samples of events do present a problem in some situations, as students may find themselves occupied when suddenly the incidents they are waiting for occurs. It is, therefore, necessary to acquaint the supervisory staff with the assignment so that their co-operation in such circumstances may be relied upon.

This method of observation can, if students are allowed such flexibility within their programme of duties, reflect the actual number of times with time intervals, that a specific aspect of behaviour takes place. If it appears, for instance, that a child is particularly withdrawn, a record could be made of any social advances made during a session. A development could indicate how many were accepted or rejected. Another, how many attempts by other children were accepted or rejected. If this type of information is required, it is sensible to compile a graph and to use coding for making the record. In this way an immediate illustration of some overall pattern or lack of it will emerge. If every time an advance was made by the child a red dot was inserted on a time plan, a black dot for rejection and a green dot for acceptance, the proportion of colour would be helpful in an initial or crude analysis.

The sparsity of red dots to begin with would confirm the tendency towards isolation. A coding which illustrated advances from other children being rejected could indicate a reluctance to participate or socialize, whereas advances consistently accepted would indicate the reverse.

One disadvantage of the event sampling method of observation is that the inexperienced may ignore other aspects of behaviour surrounding the event chosen. This can lead to events being seen in isolation, instead of against the background of the whole experience of any child. It is essential that some considerable time is spent practising the observation and recording of a wide range of typical behaviour patterns, closely linked to the study of child development.

Prepared schedules

There is a selection of charts available which catalogue the expected behaviour at ages or stages of human development. The method is to mark in some way the specific behaviour or skill acquired and at what age this takes place. A useful exercise is to compile such a document, using existing knowledge and research to outline the progressive steps anticipated. To test the validity of the document, observations should be made of a sample set of individual children of, ideally, exactly the same age for scoring. A normal distribution curve would reflect such validity (unofficially).

The Gunzburg Assessment Chart distributed through the National Society for Mentally Handicapped Children is a fascinating model of a prepared schedule. Although its completion should be made in relation to the guidelines accompanying the charts, it can be used by nursery nurses as a useful exercise in specific methodology. Even when completed in a simplified way using crude observational techniques, the result will present a diagrammatic representation of a particular behaviour pattern, showing any outstanding strengths or weaknesses or both. Finding examples of typical behaviour is not difficult. Developmental charts are published by the National Federation for Educational Research, The National Children's Bureau, and may be found in some human development publications.

As mentioned, observation of different children of the same age will provide items of typical behaviour. From this exercise a workable list could be developed to a possible idea for an assignment.

The danger of prepared schedules is that there is the possibility of the amateur becoming concerned or anxious if a child is unable to demonstrate a reasonable score. Mothers are, due to their inevitable emotional involvement, likely to take such exercises seriously. It is worth restating that the absolute norm is a textbook phenomenon. Children developing within the normal pattern are all found within the curve of normal distribution, which allows for a degree of 34 % each side of the centre. Prepared schedules are sometimes published in magazines, fortunately most emphasize the individuality and uniqueness of every child, pointing out that the schedule is simply a guide, not a diagnostic document. Though it has happened that, as a result of such checking, a mother has consulted her health visitor or doctor to discover that there is some justifiable cause for further investigation.

Illustrating identified stages

It can be a time consuming exercise illustrating stages of an identified developmental process. Either one child has to be observed over a long period of time or a selection of children of different ages have to be observed engaged in a similar activity. In the latter instance the individual assignments need to be recorded in chronological order, although the observations may be made as the suitable situation presents itself. It is, therefore, a combination of time and event sampling.

This category of observation is particularly rewarding for the student, especially if accompanied by slides, photographs, video or tape recordings or both. Whenever alternative methods of communication can be employed, learning is strengthened. The same basic principle applies, that information received through more than one sense tends to be more effective. Script, visual representation through photograph, drawing or diagram, and sound recording appeal to the intellect in a more effective way than any single vehicle of communication. Examine a written dialogue:

C   Can I have a drink?
P   Can I have a drink—what?
C   Can I have a drink of orange?

P   Can I have a drink of orange—what?
C   Orange fizzy.

Consider and compare the opportunity to see and hear the child. Not only the visual and auditory sensation but the attitude of the adult towards the child may be interpreted and probably the humour. Added to this, students will find making observations much more stimulating if they explore various methods of recording information and communicating it to others.

Useful and interesting areas on which to focus for illustrating stages of a developmental process are:

1   Playing with balloons, bricks, modelling material.
2   Feeding, dressing, toileting.
3   Climbing.
4   Illustrating a negative response.
5   Response to a stranger.
6   Asking a question for something. Tracing non-verbal/verbal communication.
7   Causes of laughter.
8   Methods of demonstrating anger.
9   Behaviour in water.
10 Drawing or painting or both.

Verbatim report

It is possible to obtain a verbatim report of a dialogue (with a real or imaginary person or toy). A group conversation, however, without a tape recorder means that only the briefest conversations may be recorded accurately.

One method is to write down all that is said, indicating by initials in the margin who has spoken. An extension is to divide the page into three columns. The first indicates time, the centre column activity, the third, speech. It is surprising how much can take place in the space of 2 to 3 minutes.

This method will present for study, a typical behaviour profile of any particular age or stage. A close scrutiny of such an observation will draw the student's attention to particular aspects which reflect the norm, or deviate from it.

Another method of handling a record of language is to write out on alternate lines the complete résumé. On the blank lines write a commentary, together with ideas on interpretation. Reference to construction should be included.

1 When rule-making seems to be illustrated: 'My dog digged a hole'.

2 When the pronoun 'me' is still used, before 'I' develops: 'Me go too'. 'Me want one'.

3 When the child attempts to hypothesize: 'I think if . . . .' 'Probably we can . . . .'

4 When feelings are expressed: 'It makes me cross when . . . .' 'I feel sad because . . . .'

Make the commentary in a different colour; it is easier to study at a later date.

An interesting exercise is to record a comparison between children whose first, or second language, is English. Does the development of English as a second language follow the same pattern as a child learning to speak naturally in his or her own tongue? If not, what is the difference and how can the child be helped to accelerate such learning? It is always sound practice to find out how a child prefers to learn or how existing learning is developing to support and strengthen, rather than confuse or negate.

Target child observation

During training it is helpful to select a particular child who deviates widely from the norm at first. This allows for the likelihood that there will be plenty of material from which to draw. Not all tutors will suggest this category of target child, preferring earlier observations to be of what may be termed 'normal children'.

What needs to be considered is the precise objective aimed for. If it is to practise recording, then the 'unusual' will present a richer vehicle for most students. If it is to study in more depth the process of human development, then, obviously children presenting relatively normal patterns are more suitable. It still remains, that when learning the skills of observation, it is helpful to work from the obvious towards the more obscure.

SELECTION

During training a child may be selected at random, whereas in a working situation there will always be a reason for such a focus. Deviant behaviour, learning problems, or even a potentially 'gifted' child all justify detailed and precise observation.

The student should be guided by the training supervisor as to which criteria, if any, to apply when making a selection. It is less than rewarding, for instance, to make a satisfactory start on an illustration of a developmental process planning to follow the same child only to find that he or she is frequently absent or likely to move away. Exceptional children do not appear often in selections of observations. It is an interesting point though, to highlight any specific area of outstanding development while matching it against other aspects. It is easier to appreciate that areas such as social and emotional development do not necessarily run parallel to that of intellect. These children deserve sensitive understanding, as they are often attempting to live up to unrealistic expectations by parents and teachers. Just as there is a tendency to expect larger children to behave in a relatively more mature manner than their average sized peers. A similar maturity in all aspects is sometimes expected of children gifted in a specific skills area.

Any of the methods mentioned may be used to make 'target' observations. A combination is also viable. Having decided on the target child, this remains the common thread, and time sampling, event sampling, development of skill, use of prepared schedule and verbatim reporting could all be used to present an integrated study.

Comparative observations

Comparative observations focus upon that which will emerge incidentally from other methods. It is a deliberate exercise aimed to present illustrations of variables reflected within the normal range of development in any given area, e.g.:

1 How does a range of 3-year-old children negotiate a simple obstacle course?

2 Compare the paintings of a set of children of exactly the same age (or as close as practicable).

3 Compare the responses of a similar set of children to the same set of questions.

4 Compare basic skills of dressing.

5 Compare responses to similar tasks of problem solving and logic.

Observations should be carried out in a variety of settings. Those made whilst in public places such as parks, shops, swimming pools, playgrounds, libraries, buses and trains will not require permission. No confidences are likely to be breached. Students are often employed on Saturdays in jobs which bring them into contact with the public and families. Such opportunities should be used, as long as job performance is not reduced. It will rarely be acceptable to make 'on the spot' notes, but the memory should hold until the evening. These observations will not have the support of explanation by skilled professionals who have direct knowledge of the child and situation, but can, nevertheless, be purposefully discussed with tutors, and in the seminar situation.

The NNEB attach much importance to the exercise of making observations; they form the fourth component scrutinized for examination purposes, along with practical and College reports and written examination results. Due to this official requirement with the overall assessment process, regulations are defined thus:

1 Observation of individual children and groups of children must form an integral part of the course throughout the 2 years.

2 Observations must be made of babies and young children throughout the age range, birth to 7 years.

3 Children must be observed in a variety of contexts, in addition to practical work placements.

4 Students must be enabled to acquire and progressively develop skills of observation, both looking and listening.

5 Students must be enabled to acquire and progressively develop a range of skills and techniques in recording observations in a variety of ways.

6 A minimum of fifty to sixty observations (including both individuals and groups) must be recorded by the end of the course.

7 Every student must present a file of observations as part of the final examination.

8 All observation files will be presented for scrutiny by the external examiners. These examiners select a sample of files and pay special attention to the work of candidates recommended for failure and all those classed as borderline candidates.

Now that the written examination consists of multiple choice and essay type questions, the total assessment pattern continues as one of the fairest and most comprehensive within the qualifying system.

Chapter 13
The Nursery Nurse in Different Roles

The NNEB Certificate is the passport into a wide variety of employment situations. It is recognized by employers within education, social services and health authority establishments as well as by private employers. The qualified nursery nurses consequently find themselves the holders of a variety of titles: Nursery Assistant, Welfare Assistant, Nursery Officer, Houseparent, Play Therapist, Nanny, Nursery Governess or Assistant Matron have all been used, as well as Nursery Nurse.

During the 2 year course most students will have the opportunity to experience a wide variety of settings which concentrate on the care, health and education of young children. Within such a programme it is hoped that students will include the category of children deemed to have special needs. Obviously each individual experience or period of training will necessarily be of a relatively short duration. Each part, however, will act as a diagnostic tool, as well as form a valuable training/education component within a total programme.

It is not expected, or desirable, that the newly qualified nursery nurses should hope to be fully efficient in any single area. They will develop a good working knowledge of a number of areas of practice and be ready to decide in which of these their strengths and commitments lie. At this point their learning finds new direction and depth. This is not always recognized, especially when newly qualified staff become responsible for a family group. Due to staff shortages in specific geographical areas it is accepted that this may be unavoidable but, however diligent and supportive the senior staff, it is not an ideal situation.

The children in day nurseries frequently come from families already coping with a variety of social, emotional, physical, intellectual or moral needs which are partly or wholly unmet. Any stresses caused are likely to affect the total family structure, most of all the vulnerable members who are the children. These children in day care, cannot be nurtured in isolation, and a mature sensitivity and understanding of family dynamics is critically important for effective therapeutic support. A development from such support, would be progress towards establishment or re-establishment of family stability. As children are such a valuable component of any unit, the approach to their care ought to be, not only of high quality, but administered by mature, sensitive, experienced practitioners. Newly qualified nursery nurses are not fully equipped yet to carry this responsibility. They are ready to learn.

COMMUNICATION

With parents

Whether in the role of friend, adviser, authority figure or target, communication with parents is a vital component in the field of effective child care. Sometimes it is a pleasure, sometimes it is a stressful task.

The dominant influence, in the particular role adopted, will depend both on the specific environment and on the situation. The nursery nurse, for example, working in the family situation is more unlikely to adopt an authoratitive role with a parent than a colleague in Social Services. On the other hand it would be reasonable to expect that a qualified nursery nurse would experience a variety of roles within most of the work situations traditionally entered.

Accepting this, such personnel need to be mature, well-informed, confident without dominating and, most of all, sensitive to other people's feelings both positive and negative. There are those who go through life without developing this sensitivity. Such people often make better speakers than listeners. Listening to others is a skill which does not come naturally to all, and there may often be justification for learning and practising in order to be able to encourage those in need, to express themselves adequately. Expression and body language convey messages indicating receptiveness, interest and understanding, or impatience, distraction and boredom. A useful book to study is *Manwatching* by Desmond Morris. Such non-verbal communication can directly influence the nature of a dialogue, and consequently the outcome may at times differ widely from that intended.

Establishing a dialogue

One of the prime objectives when considering communication with parents must be that of establishing a useful dialogue. Listening is equally important, if not more so, than speaking. There is often a tendency to feel ill at ease during short silences within a conversation and, consequently, there is a great temptation to fill such gaps, whether or not it is appropriate to do so. Such breaks in conversation can be most positive. The speaker has the opportunity to organize his or her thoughts and reflect, feeling what is being said must be of value and worth. The listener strengthens the relationship by conveying such a message and goes further towards achieving the speaker's objective. Another benefit is that an anxious participant, probably the parent, will feel able to contribute more as he or she feels the acceptance of the listener—in this instance the nursery nurse.

Never appear to be waiting to make a remark or comment; this has an adverse effect on the person who is finding it difficult to transmit his or her real anxieties or problems. It may happen that two or three encounters take place before the *real* problems are expressed. During the first one or two meetings a testing takes place, before sufficient trust is established for the cosmetics to be removed or dispensed with. Only then can the encounter reflect true communication; only then can problem-solving commence.

Parents should always be made welcome in the nursery (Fig. 13.1). Children with families should not be considered apart from them. Their families influence them more than any other agency throughout their experience. Therefore care or treatment or both should follow a programme which incorporates an awareness of the home situation, together with an appropriate participation by the adult or adults primarily responsible for the child.

It may be appropriate to recommend minimum attendance by the responsible person at a day nursery or similar establishment, in order to observe good child care practice. On the other hand, it may

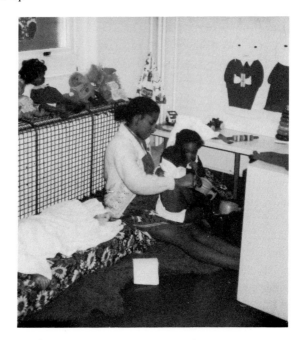

Fig. 13.1　A mother plays with her children in the nursery.

be advisable to request the parent to adopt certain practices to extend and support a programme. This could apply to children who are disturbed, handicapped, injured, sick, or displaying specific learning difficulties. Such a partnership can only be anticipated as a result of effective communication. The benefits of such partnerships beg no further justification.

Parents who present a need for support may fall into certain categories. The young, the isolated, the immigrant, the handicapped, those of low intelligence, those with low incomes, the single parent, those with handicapped children or a large family close in age, are among the parents who, at some stage, will almost certainly need support. This support will vary from the kind offered by a close relative or friend to specialized counselling.

What is often not appreciated is that help and support is always available. Knowing which way to turn is the first vital item of knowledge which should be made available to all mothers. Maybe telephone directories should carry this information in a similar section as that ascribed to hospitals. Libraries and clinics are sometimes alien places to the mothers in most need, yet these centres are often the only source of basic contact information.

AREAS OF PRACTICE

Within education

According to local policy, nursery nurses are employed in nursery units or classes, infant classes, special units, special schools and children's centres. The children's centres are staffed and administered jointly between education and social services with other facilities provided by the health authority on the premises. Classes in schools always have their own teacher who determines teaching method and implementation, under the overall authority held by the Headmistress or Headmaster.

A nursery nurse will usually be employed where it is considered that there is a special need. The children may be in very large groups, be under the age of 5, the school may be found in a designated educational priority area (EPA). There may be a policy of integration for handicapped pupils, or the school may come within the definition of a special school. Such schools cater for the needs of physically or mentally handicapped children or for those emotionally disturbed. In any case, the *Nursery Assistant*, as she or he will be called, certainly has plenty to do.

It depends on the individual teacher how much responsibility will be carried, but many happy partnerships emerge which are of maximum benefit to the children.

Routine duties ascribed to the assistant will include: care, preparation and maintenance of the environment inside and out. This does not mean heavy cleaning or gardening, but day-to-day light cleaning, keeping tidy and watching for broken or dangerous toys or equipment. It also means displaying a developed awareness by presenting a suitable environment for the particular group of children cared for. It means preparing the room for the morning, and offering a variety of activities, as well as rearranging furniture at times and changing displays, pictures and posters to stimulate fresh interest.

Basic materials and tools may be the responsibility of the nursery assistant. Clay, dough, paints, glue need to be stored with care, refilled or replaced, and ready to use in a safe, clean, workable condition. Pencils need to be sharpened, books repaired and jig-saws kept together and complete. Pets need to be well cared for and sensibly handled by the children, under supervision.

Basic skills learned by the children under the guidance of the teacher need to be practised—sometimes it seems endlessly—to achieve acceptable levels. Nursery assistants are the watching eyes, listening ears and providers of well-informed advice and encouragement. They are the substitute mothers when a child needs extra support in situations of stress, illness or injury. With more than 20 small children to look after, even one, needing individual attention can create a problem, and during any single day this situation is likely to emerge more than once or twice. Nursery nurses, as a result of their training, are well prepared to communicate with the child, displaying a special need for comfort, reassurance, encouragement, and time to be listened to. Their skills of observation are also an invaluable tool with which they can support the teacher.

Most nursery nurses demonstrate special personal skills. They may be musical, artistic, or have an aptitude for telling or dramatizing stories. Sensible teachers will ensure that both adult and children benefit from such resources. Nursery assistants may accept responsibility for a craft or painting area. They may plan and maintain a book corner, holding a regular story time. They may prepare and carry out cooking sessions, knowing the opportunities for a range of learning which such activities present. They may develop a music corner and plan a related selection of activities. Physical skills in water and on dry land can be practised and improved with the support of a good nursery nurse assistant.

It is worth restating that the nursery nurses are qualified people and if welcomed as team members can contribute much to the life of any school. Their duties will vary. In a school for the physically handicapped there will be many routine caring tasks which are unnecessary in an infants' school, just as in a nursery class or unit there will be proportionally more 'mothering' required than in a top infants' class.

It is becoming more unusual to find a nursery nurse in an ordinary infants' school, unless handicapped children are integrated. To offer teachers some support, the nursery nurse may sometimes be 'shared' on a rota basis. One disadvantage of this arrangement is that relationships will be relatively transitory. One advantage is that some activities may be followed which would otherwise be impossible to organize by the teacher alone. Activities such as cooking, shopping, and sewing, would probably fall into this category.

Young teachers may be unfamiliar with the training or education of nursery nurses and be unaware of their particular role and value within the classroom and school life generally. The local or closest college offering an NNEB course would normally provide informative and helpful guidance.

Policy will vary from one authority to another with reference to the employment of nursery nurses in their establishments. There is no national rule and it is unlikely that this will emerge in the foreseeable future. It should be noted that for some 'special schools', the vacancy advertized may require a welfare assistant. The job description, however, will be very closely related to that of nursery assistant.

Within social services

Nursery officer is the name now given to nursery nurses working in social services establishments, usually day nurseries or centres. Similarly, in place of Matron, and Deputy or Assistant, we find Officer in Charge or Deputy Officer in Charge, affectionately known as OICs and DOICs. It is possible to become an OIC as an NNEB certificate holder but many have now studied further courses, such as the Certificate in Social Services or Certificate of Qualification in Social Work. Others are initially trained or educated as teachers or nurses.

Nursery officers will either find themselves in partnership situations jointly responsible for a family group, or a group of children within a specific age span, or solely responsible in a similar capacity. These systems are known as vertical and horizontal grouping respectively. In either case the officers will act as surrogate mothers for the children in their group. The ratio of adult to child is usually 1 : 4; the number of staff qualified or experienced or both will depend on the geographical area.

It is difficult in some of the more deprived areas to attract staff of a high calibre who will offer stability to a nursery by remaining in the post for a reasonable period of time. The hours of duty and lack of school holidays means that few mature people are found in the day nursery situation, leaving most of the responsibility to newly qualified and young staff.

The daily routine in a nursery has become progressively more flexible in an attempt to meet more directly the changing needs within the society it serves. Not all children come at the same time, nor do they all leave together. Some may come for a day or two each week, allowing an overstressed mother some respite, others to learn to communicate in English as a preparation for school. Handicapped children come to allow mother to relax and have some precious free time, and to experience the stimulation and friendship of able-bodied companions.

CHILDREN'S NEEDS

If the broad areas of children's needs are identified it will become clear how demanding are the everyday tasks of nursery officers.

Physical needs

Nursery officers will prepare suitable environments offering opportunity for safe challenge and exploration, thus encouraging the search for learning, together with practice of muscular development towards refined control. They will be familiar with expected stages of growth and development, enabling them to plan programmes of activities aiming towards the next progressive step for the individual within a group situation. Due to this familiarity, and the skills of observation they will be able to detect any sign indicating deviation from the norm. As a result of considerable practice they can record any signs and symptoms which will help the specialist practitioner to make an informed diagnosis.

Nursery nurses will be able to handle any minor illnesses and administer first aid after almost any of the accidents which may occur during a routine day. They will be able to consider the normal dietary requirements of the average child and make a broad analysis of whether or not that child's needs are being met during the day. The difficulty sometimes arises when the child is inadequately nourished at home. This can arise for various reasons, such as contrasting cultural habits, severe financial hardship or simple ignorance. During the time in the nursery special dietary needs can also be catered for and the mother helped, if necessary, to continue the pattern at home.

Clothing is not the direct responsibility of the nursery officer in a day care situation but help can be given. If the child is unsuitably clothed a sensitive approach to the mother can achieve results. Immigrant families often take some time to adapt properly to unfamiliar climatic conditions and the children may not be provided with suitable clothing for quite some time. Mothers living under poor physical conditions and suffering from stress, may delay washing clothes, reaching the point where they are hygienically a hazard. Such a situation requires an extra sensitive approach. Simply washing the clothes at the nursery, although it solves the immediate problem, does not alleviate the underlying cause which may be one deserving specialized attention.

The other basic physical need is for rest, for the child's sake, not for the convenience of the nursery staff, or 'tidiness' of the routine. Each individual child requires a different amount of rest and sleep and a flexible day allows for this. Rest and sleep should always be a pleasure, and children ought to be brought up to regard it in this way. Sadly this does not happen in many cases. It can still be observed in some nurseries that children are too strongly persuaded to go to sleep. Bed is still used by parents as a form of punishment.

To sum up, the areas within the term physical provision are fresh air, food and clothing, with safe suitable exercise for body and mind. In adequate supply these will prevent most illnesses and accidents. If any do occur, initial treatment is part of the responsibility of the nursery officer.

One last word on physical provision is an important reference to physical contact. All young things in order to thrive, need love and security expressed by means of physical affection. Some children are deprived of such contact and need holding and cuddling more than others. Sadly there is often an expressed fear of 'spoiling', when a child demands such comfort. Maybe a little too much, rather than too little is a calculated risk worth taking.

Social needs

Nursery officers will by setting good examples encourage socially acceptable behaviour. Direct example is one of the most effective teaching methods and obvious instruction is less productive. This is not always as easy as it sounds, the nursery officers may at times be guilty of expecting the children to 'do as I say' rather than 'do as I do'.

To socialize, communication is the main vehicle; language development and practice is vitally important. It means listening to children as much as, if not more than, speaking to them. Nursery officers need to give individual attention when possible and 'divide themselves' fairly. During many activities such as eating meals, playing games, or listening to stories, there is opportunity to develop socially acceptable patterns of behaviour.

Emotional needs

Nursery officers will be adopting the roles of 'surrogate mother' and therefore by implication be emotionally involved. They should elicit trust and affection from the children in their care and the children, in return, should be able to rely on them as dependable, consistent, caring adults. Within these few words lies a very demanding role for the nursery officer.

Intellectual needs

Due to the nursery officers' knowledge of human development, they will need to plan activities with regard to the ages and stages of the children in their group. These will have to match the children's abilities and aptitudes, taking into consideration the next stage aimed towards. They will also need to perceive when a stage has been successfully negotiated in order to present fresh challenges. Knowledge of basic skills will enable them to prepare the children for more formalized learning on entering the school situation.

Setting of values

Children develop a sense of right and wrong naturally, by example and through direct instruction. Once it is accepted that there is no clear black and white distinction in the area of human moral values, the complexity of their development is easier to appreciate.

Children will normally acquire the values held by their parents and hold to these throughout life, even though demonstrating some deviation, usually in adolescence. It is commonly accepted that children reach the age of reason and moral responsibility at about the age of seven. It is therefore more realistic to see a guiding role at preschool age more closely related to responsible, acceptable social behaviour, as opposed to the development of moral values. Good and bad, right or wrong are merely words, not established concepts.

This illustrates the challenges faced by nursery officers when they plan their programmes with a view to meeting the needs expressed or anticipated, by the children in their care.

DAILY ROUTINE

The vehicle through which nursery officers aim to meet needs may appear as follows:

8.30- 9.30 am	Reception of children. Hot drink and toast, breakfast for those who need it.
9.30-10.30 am	Free play, followed by planned group activity (toileting).
10.30-11.00 am	Outside play whenever practicable.
11.00-11.30 am	Drink. Quiet time, story or play.
11.30-11.45 am	Prepare for lunch (toileting).

11.45-12.30 pm	Lunch (toileting).
12.30- 2.00 pm	Rest, sleep or quiet play (toileting).
2.00- 3.00 pm	Free play (partly outside when suitable) or organized group activity.
3.15 pm	Tea.
3.30 pm	Story, finger rhymes.
4.00 pm	Free play.
4.30 pm	Children start going home.
5.00 pm	Television if suitable.

Routine toiletting should be flexibly applied.

Within health authority establishments

Nursery nurses will be found working in maternity units, children's wards, assessment centres and hospital staff nurseries or crèches.

MATERNITY UNITS

In maternity units or wards the role of the nursery nurse is twofold. Firstly, to assist in the care of the new-born baby, either full-term or preterm; secondly to help and support the mothers during the first few days after confinement.

Most babies are born healthy and strong, and soon establish a satisfactory pattern of feeding and sleeping, and thus present few problems. According to the practice in any individual maternity unit, the new-borns will spend a certain proportion of time in the nursery and the remainder close to their mothers. As has already been emphasized, it is crucial that separation from the moment of birth is kept at a minimum in order that emotional bonding takes place. Such bonding is thought to have considerable effect on future relationships with the mother and, as a direct result, with other human beings too. Individuals who are unable to relate satisfactorily and appropriately as they mature may well suffer throughout life. Such people are almost always sad, unhappy individuals.

To allow the mother the maximum opportunity to rest, it is likely that babies will stay in the nursery during the night, although this is not always the case. During this time the nursery nurse will take care of the baby's needs, except when a mother is breastfeeding and herself needs to feed her baby. When the milk supply is becoming established the breasts may well be too uncomfortable, if left for more than 3-4 hours. Once again, all people are individuals and many mothers may not have this problem.

So, during the night, routine care, feeding, changing and observing of all babies will be the responsibility of nursing staff. If there is any cause for concern, then medical expertise is available at a moments notice. During the night the new-born who need special care, either through illness, physical or mental defect, or prematurity, will receive more specialized routine attention and similar observation through human and technological means.

The nursery nurse will learn to carry out many of these procedures. Most of the routine in maternity units follows a relatively similar pattern during the day too; the difference being that, when the mother is awake, she not only shares the responsibility for her own child, but according to her ability and previous experience will take over such responsibility. In this way, when she is ready to go home, her confidence will have been established whilst in a safe, secure environment.

Although nursery nurses may not have experienced childbirth and breastfeeding themselves it is part of their role to advise and support the inexperienced mothers during the first few days after confinement. They therefore need to observe sensitive and experienced nursing staff carrying out such roles in a caring and effective way. After a certain amount of such observing and learning, they will be ready to assume such a responsibility on their own, or without direct support.

BATHING THE NEWLY BORN BABY

One of the tasks which seems to elicit most apprehension from new mothers is that of bathing the new baby. She is afraid of losing hold, letting the cord stump become wet and of hurting him or her.

The nursery nurse will demonstrate more than once if necessary, before encouraging the mother to carry out the procedure herself.

Preparation

Assemble everything that is required:
Bath, e.g. a baby bath, an adaptor for an adult bath, or a high sink/ bath, a suitable polythene bowl.

Jug	Zinc and caster oil cream or
Cotton wool	petroleum jelly
Soap	Towel
Baby shampoo	Clean clothes
Powder	Nappies

Covered bucket for soiled napkins and receptacle for discarded swabs.

Make sure the required bottlefeed is prepared if necessary. If breastfeeding, the mother should be ready, that is, clean herself and place fresh gauze pads inside her bra. It is a little awkward sometimes because this stimulation may cause the milk to 'rush in'. This happens naturally and for the first few seconds can be so fast and copious that the baby has difficuly in beginning to feed. The general preparation for feeding can cause this flow even before the baby starts to suck. It is interesting to note that, if breastfeeding, even thinking about feeding one's own baby can cause the milk to flow.

The mother or nurse (although reference will be to either, nurse will be used for brevity) should wear clean protection, a wipe-clean oilcloth or PVC apron is suitable, ideally covered with a towelling protection for comfort and to prevent the baby slipping on the knee. All utensils should be clean, the room should be warm and the bathing area free from draughts.

Half fill the baby bath, or other suitable receptacle, and prepare the water either hotter or colder than eventually required. The temperature should be comfortable to the elbow. Have a jug of cool or hot water accordingly to ensure correct temperature. This avoids moving around after the first procedure is completed which takes a few minutes depending on the expertise of the nurse.

Procedure

The first step is washing the baby's face and head, paying special attention to the eyes. While this is happening, talk and laugh with the baby.

Undress the baby, leaving on the nappy and wrap him or her in a towel swaddling the whole body. Using a fresh cotton wool swab for each eye, wipe gently from the centre once and discard the swab. This avoids any foreign body or infection being introduced. Likewise, gently clean the nostrils with cotton wool pulled into tiny points, then the ears. *Never* use cotton buds or home-made tools fashioned out of cotton wool and cocktail sticks; these are rigid and can cause damage, especially if the baby makes a sudden movement. Clean only as far as can be seen, is a safe rule.

If the head is to be washed, dampen, then apply a little shampoo to the hand and massage gently all over the head, paying special attention to the fontanelle, this is not as delicate as is sometimes supposed by a new mother. Some prefer to reverse these two procedures—head and hair before the face. Hold the baby comfortably and securely over the bath and thoroughly rinse the head, drying gently either with a small towel or part of the large one wrapped round the baby.

Remove the nappy, cleanse the area thoroughly of any faeces. Next, place the baby face down and soap the back, quickly and thoroughly. Turning the baby over onto his or her back, soap again, making sure creases and folds are covered. Lift the baby as shown by the experts—using the right or left hand support the head and shoulders and grasp under the arm furthest away, holding it in the most comfortable position. The other hand will hold the lower limbs. Make sure the left-hander is arranged so that she can reach everything and has access to the bath in a natural position.

Release the hold on the legs or ankles once the baby is in the bath and allow him or her some time to enjoy. Splash the water over the baby and continue to talk and laugh. On lifting the baby out on to the towel (either on the knee or on a flat surface, whichever is preferred) he or she may cry. By wrapping securely in the towel, he or she will become dry as a result of cuddling and patting. Open the towel and gently attend to any skin folds and creases, especially in the neck, behind the ears, under the arms, behind the knees and in the genital area. If appropriate, treat the cord stump as directed, probably swabbing, drying and dusting with medicated powder.

After ensuring that the baby is completely dry, lotion, oil or powder may be applied sparingly, especially the powder which must never be used as a drying agent. Apply the usual protection to the nappy area and put on a clean, warm, aired nappy, then plastic pants. These pants only cause problems if they are used to avoid changing nappies, as often as necessary. Dress the baby and settle down to feed him or her in a cosy environment. This is one of the most rewarding and emotionally satisfying times of the day.

The baby will usually be happy to settle down after feeding and the clearing up can be carried out. If the baby is content to wait and watch the cleaning up before he or she is fed, this is sometimes preferred. Make sure the baby is never left, even for a minute or two, unless he or she is safe and secure.

WITHIN CHILDREN'S WARDS AND HOSPITALS

Nursery nurses will be found in children's wards and hospitals. Their role is to offer the children emotional support, and to present them with activities appropriate to their age, stage and particular illness. This diagnosis is essential, as children's needs, other than of a physical nature, are equally affected by illness. They usually regress intellectually, their powers of concentration and levels of patience are diminished. Therefore, activities often need to match an earlier stage of development than the child's chronological age would suggest.

Knowledge of normal development, together with skills of observation, help the good nursery nurses to present suitable programmes for the children. They also have to take into account that medical treatment will take priority and their plans must be flexible. Also, that according to various treatments, the child's attitude and ability will vary from day to day.

Provision will also vary from a well-stocked playroom closely related to a small nursery classroom, to a couple of boxes of toys. Sometimes an enthusiastic nursery nurse will be able to build up a good selection of basic materials necessary for the effective stimulation of the children, almost from scratch. Normally maximum support is received from those in the position of providing such resources.

AS PLAY THERAPISTS

Nursery nurses in the role of play therapists do not normally wear a uniform. This helps to identify them in an informal role, although they are a real part of the hospital team. Children who, unfortunately, sometimes have to endure unpleasant treatment, need to relate confidently to staff such as nursery nurses who are not involved in the administration of medical procedures. This may seem unfair to the nurses but it is a fact that, after stressful experiences, children understandably do often regard a uniform with apprehension. The nursery nurses are able to act as surrogate mothers, they hopefully have the time and the skill to communicate effectively with children in need of emotional support.

If a long hospital stay is necessary, and this is becoming increasingly rare except where there is no real alternative, arrangements will be made for the children to continue their education. In most cases there are teachers specially appointed, who attempt to cover programmes for a very wide range of age and ability. They will also have special knowledge and regard for the extra stress that illness and treatment can cause and the effect it will have on the capacity for and the attitude towards learning.

Even very sick children whose prognosis is poor will be found workng hard on their 'school' lessons and assignments. Obviously no undue pressure is ever applied, but it has been found that children are usually very keen to continue formal learning; it may well serve to strengthen links with 'normality'.

Children who are admitted to hospital in need of care and protection, officially 'at risk', or suffering from non-accidental injury, may benefit considerably if there are nursery nurses on the staff. Much of their care will not be specifically medical but of emotional, social or intellectual repair and rebuilding. Such children may not have successfully passed the accepted milestones of development and will need to be guided through them systematically and with considerable skill and understanding.

Some of the saddest children are those who have not learned to laugh. Some of the most rewarding moments are sharing laughter with these children after long patient hours of encouragement and tender, loving care (TLC). Working with babies and children in the hospital environment is probably one of the jobs offering more scope for variety and demonstration of a wider range of skills than may at first be appreciated.

Added to those mentioned, there are also many hospitals offering day care facilities for outpatients and members of staff. Nursery nurses in this situation will work in very much the same way as the nursery officer in a local authority day nursery. Duties involved are illustrated in the specimen job description (Fig. 13.2). There will, however, be one main difference in that almost all children will attend according to parental shift patterns or treatment programmes. Planning activities will need to take this into account, especially with regard to special treats or parties so that all children have the opportunity to participate as far as possible.

Nursery nurses in any of the situations mentioned are normally employed by the health authority, although the day care facilities may come under the jurisdiction of the social services department in some aspects.

Private employment

There are many certificated nursery nurses employed in private households as nannies. According to the conditions of service, the title 'mother's help' or nursery governess may be used. It is essential that the employee in such situations establishes with the employer, prior to commencing work, a very clear understanding about duties, salary, responsibility, social position, time off-duty, insurance and terms of notice. There are no legal guidelines and little legal protection.

Having said this, there are hundreds of very happy and successful arrangements made every year through advertisements and by personal contacts. There are also various agencies which offer to intro-

Fig. 13.2 Specimen Job Description—Staff Nursery Nurse

Responsible to: Day Nursery Matron or Officer in Charge

Reports to: Day Nursery Matron

Overall Duty: To provide day-to-day care for children attending the Nursery

Specific Duties
(A) General:
1. To develop an assuring relationship with the children being cared for.
2. To provide extra individual attention to children during their first few weeks of attendance at the Nursery.
3. To provide a varied and stimulating environment in which the children may develop their basic skills.
4. To observe the children and report to the Matron or Assistant Matron any signs of illness or distress.
5. To supervise meals and toilet routine.
6. To care for the children's personal and Nursery clothes.
7. To maintain a careful watch over children and report anything that may prove a hazard to the safety of children or staff.
8. To create a happy and relaxed atmosphere in which the children spend their day.
9. To develop a reassuring relationship with parents.
10. To assist with the care and cleanliness of all Nursery equipment and to report to the Matron, or Assistant Matron, any damage or deficiency.

(B) Care of Babies:
1. To be responsible for preparation of feeds, the sterilization of feed-making equipment and liaison with parents on babies' feeding schedules.
2. To be responsible for the care and cleanliness of all baby room equipment including prams for outdoor use.
3. To prepare older babies for transition to Toddler Group.
4. To ensure that all baby room equipment is in a safe condition for use, and to report any fault to the Matron or Assistant Matron.

(C) Care of Toddlers:
1. To toilet train children, and encourage younger children to feed themselves.
2. To provide play facilities allowing for needs of the age group.
3. To prepare older toddlers for transition to older age group.

(D) Care for Older Children:
1. To provide varied opportunities for play.
2. To train children to care for toys, books, and other items; to encourage them to help with simple tasks, to teach them to share and to accept discipline.
3. To encourage independence in older children prior to them starting to attend school.

All Staff Nursery Nurses help in the training of Nursery Nurse Students, and are also responsible for sharing their duties with Nursery Assistants.

All Nursery Staff must comply at all times with the regulations in respect of Health & Safety at Work.

duce suitable families to prospective nannies or mother's helps. It is difficult to recommend one more than another; the best method is to follow personal recommendations, always read the small print and ask for advice from tutors, parents and, if in serious doubt, even a solicitor before signing anything.

In addition to the qualification of the NNEB Certificate, various extra skills may be asked for, such as affection for horses or dogs, or the ability to swim or drive. It is becoming increasingly common for a nonsmoker to be mentioned. Even apart from these criteria, the range of skills required in order to be a successful nannie is very broad. Among these will be found cooking, laundering, ironing, care of the environment, entertaining, first aid, care of the sick child, and competence to assume full responsibility if the parents wish to go away. Incidentally, any cooking, laundering or light housework should only be in connection with the nannie or children, other than when employed as a mother's help when duties are usually of a more general nature.

One of the problems frequently associated with this category of employment is that of isolation and loneliness. More often than not the nannie is well-accommodated and has the benefit of facilities such as a television or even the use of the car. She may well accompany the family on holidays abroad. This often sounds glamorous but enjoying such 'treats' is not quite the same for an employee, who is obliged to follow her duties, especially in the evening whilst the parents go out and socialize.

A pattern of working as a daily nannie seems to be gaining popularity. The nursery nurses may carry on their own private lives and the family may continue to enjoy their privacy too. Fewer and fewer families now live in properties large enough to accommodate living-in staff but more and more mothers are returning to work, hence the emergence of the daily nannie.

Nannie sharing, although not common, is also an arrangement some families have found successful. The nannie will care for children from two families, either together or on a rota basis. In the former situation the children will spend the time in one house, in the latter the nannie will be shared between two homes. The benefits are obvious, the children have company and parents are able to work, even on a part-time basis, without the financial burden of a full-time nannie.

It may seem that there are more problems associated with private employment than any other. This is not necessarily the case but it is advisable to consider very carefully many more aspects before making a decision. Living within a family situation demands a flexible and tolerant attitude from all concerned. It is also vital that the various personalities involved are able to work and live harmoniously together. Sometimes it takes a little time to establish whether or not such harmony will develop. There should be a period during which either employer or employee may choose to discontinue the arrangement, without any unpleasantness on either side.

A scan through a couple of the weekly publications which contain a situations vacant section will provide a good illustration of the nature of vacancies currently available. The ambition to work as a private nannie is not uncommon and many young women spend happy and rewarding years with families with whom they remain in contact for generations.

Other related areas

Added to the categories mentioned, nursery nurses may be found in other less familiar situations. There is a small team working at a London airport caring for children who have time to spend in between flights. There are hostesses for children in holiday camps and family hotels. There are nursery nurses fostering and acting as childminders. There is a very small number acting as hostesses on cruise ships, although most of these posts are now held by mature qualified teachers. There are a number of industrial crèches staffed by nursery nurses; also facilities temporarily provided at large exhibitions or trade fairs, and at Wimbledon during the Tennis Championships.

A nursery nurse can prove a very capable manageress, after further training, of a store retailing babies' or children's wear or both, toys and other related items. Dental surgeons who work with children find nursery nurses make very good chairside assistants. Further training opportunities attract a small proportion of graduates every year, some into nursing, others towards teaching after working for the requisite A-levels. Social work interests some, but to qualify experience must first be gained in order to negotiate sponsorship. Information about those who may follow such a path is very limited.

PRACTICAL TRAINING

Nursery nurses who receive adequate career advice and successfully qualify, provide children with care of the highest quality and integrity today. Part of their success is that they know they are fulfilling their ambition in a highly skilled way having had the benefit of a most comprehensive training and education programme. The quality of this programme is largely dependent on the supervision of the student during the practical placement.

Working with students

During their 2 year period in college and practical training establishment, students must negotiate various hurdles. One which presents more problems than it should, is the relationship between the learner and those responsible for facilitating the learning experience. Nursery staff recently qualified seem to forget very quickly what it feels like to be new, apprehensive and nervous about the unknown. It is true that the age difference between the two may be minimal and the disparity between roles is substantial. Some maturity is needed to handle this type of situation but development varies considerably with the individual.

LEARNING BY EXAMPLE

A recommendation for special responsibility should be assigned to those who have most to offer in a learning situation. It is not simply the best model, it is a combination of skills. Amongst these one would hope to find:

1 First class child care practice.
2 Ability to communicate in an effective way, at all levels, including listening.
3 Perception about other people's unstated feelings.

4 Interest in learning as a process.
5 A desire to be involved in such processes in a responsible role.
6 Motivation for further learning.
7 Ability to adapt happily to a variety of personalities.
8 Flexibility.
9 Enough confidence and maturity to accept that some students are going to be more able in some specific cases than oneself.

STUDENT INVOLVEMENT

It is useful to remember small things, such as greeting the students each day—it is nice to be noticed. Include them in conversation during periods in the staff room. There is nothing worse than the feeling of isolation and rejection engendered by being ignored. Likewise, in the group room or classroom, avoid carrying on dialogues with other staff members about trivia related to private and social life or other members of staff. This is unprofessional practice, but there is a tendency for it to become a fairly familiar activity in some establishments. The students become understandably embarrassed but, more importantly, it presents to them a model with which they identify in a negative way. Students' expections of nursery nurses are high; they are impressionable and easily disillusioned.

Do not make a habit of giving the student the routine, boring or unpleasant jobs. It is true that they need to appreciate that such chores are an essential and integral part of child care. It is unfair, however, to expect them to perform them more often than is necessary to acquire the skill and knowledge to be responsible for such procedures in the future.

Students are not paid, quite the reverse in many cases as they are fee-paying. Once any activity has ceased to be of value in a learning role, it should no longer be repeated unless some specific situation causes this to be necessary. Most activities with the children, even if seeming to be repetitive, are never truly so. A small group, for example, may engage in cooking on a weekly basis. Such a job is so rich in experiences that the planner will appreciate this and ensure that extensions to existing skills and knowledge are organized as well as allowing for re-inforcement of those already introduced.

It must be appreciated that alongside intended learning outcomes is a vast fund of individual learning unique to each child. This is often forgotten, rarely elicited and hardly ever tested. The value of such learning should never be underrated. This principle applies to the package of knowledge, skills and attitudes acquired by the student nursery nurses. They take away with them, as part of that package, a store of components hidden from those who plan their programmes. The positive elements must heavily outweigh the negative if the qualification is to maintain the existing image.

Guidelines for training

Students will require certain needs to be met by those directly involved in their general training. These will vary with the individual, some needing more support than others. It should be noted that there is little relationship between the amount of help initially required by any student, and her eventual performance. It is necessary to avoid judging before the student is sufficiently settled to display abilities and attitudes which may more realistically reflect her potential.

Most students are coping with a complex set of demands: leaving school, starting college, leaving friends, making new friends, being part of the staff rather than a pupil, and having more responsibility for an academic programme. Adjustments are all necessary in order to work in a satisfactory way in the practical training establishment. The person responsible for any student needs to be carefully chosen. He or she must be mature enough to empathise with a young learner, and be eager and able to communicate the skills required in any given situation.

Clearly some skills cannot be practised, but should be observed by the student. Every opportunity must be given for observation as this is a vital aspect of learning. Such job experience would include being present at medical examinations, participating in communicating with parents presenting special needs, taking part in decision-making, and sometimes attending case conferences and court hearings.

PRACTICAL SKILLS

Skills which require practice and a degree of competence to be demonstrated include:

1 Planning, preparation, care and maintenance of the environment, indoors, and outside.

2 Matching of the environment to the age and ability of the children.

3 Selection, provision and appropriate administration of nourishment to children catering for each age group.

4 Attention to hygiene and presentation of food.

5 Understanding some of the problems commonly encountered in relation to food.

6 Reference to the diets of ethnic groups.

7 Appreciation of the need for adequate rest and sleep for the different age groups, and the need for provision to be made for this indoors and outside.

8 Special reference to some practices of persuading young children to sleep.

9 Knowledge of development of control of body functions linked to routine care and guidance, with attention to hygiene.

10 Sensitive handling of children especially during toddler period when some independence is normally displayed.

11 Demonstration of appropriate level of language to be used according to chronological and/or developmental age.

12 Opportunity to observe communication between professionals, e.g. health visitors, social workers, and local authority representatives.

13 Introduction to formal report writing, purposeful record keeping and observations.

14 Demonstration of knowledge of normal child development linked to adequate provision and proper use of resources, natural and manufactured, either purpose built or adapted.

15 Sensitive handling of play situations shown by knowing when to participate and support or extend, or keep a watching eye and observe.

IN SCHOOL

The student will act as support to the teacher in school and at the same time share her gifts and talents with the children. If appropriate, the nursery nurse can be responsible for groups engaged in art, craft or musical activities or areas in which she feels confident. She should never be used to perform routine tasks during her training period, at the expense of extending learning opportunities, or observing the children. One of the most valuable roles the nursery nurse can adopt is that of individual support or comfort.

IN THE DAY NURSERY

The student is preparing to adopt a role of considerable responsibility and will need to be competent in a wide range of activities within the day nursery. Special note should be taken of initiative, maturity and sensitivity. Reports should always indicate any potential for an unsupervised, responsible role. If, for any reason, a placement does not proceed satisfactorily, it is fair, after discussion, to offer the student alternative opportunity to succeed. Conflicts of personality do occur, and it is in the interests of all concerned, especially the children, that they should be afforded a stable and happy environment.

Fortunately for most students the training period is happy and constructive, for which all those who share the responsibility should be thanked.

Clearly the NNEB certificate is a most flexible qualification, recognized on a world-wide basis. However, it does have limitations, the main one being that, at present, there is no obvious path through which the Certificate holder can achieve more advanced qualifications and achieve higher status and responsibility, without commencing on the bottom rung of another ladder. There are a few exceptions but these are sufficiently rare to be negligible.

Chapter 14
The Technological Age

It is likely that the children being cared for and educated in nurseries and infant schools today will grow up into a world changed through the technological developments already influencing our life. To make some real attempt to prepare them, it is necessary for adults to accelerate their own rate of familiarisation and education.

Physical communication has become more and more a means to an end. Technology has reduced the time spent in transit, at the expense of pleasure in many instances. It is therefore useful to explore the positive experiences encountered through any method of travel. Whenever possible aim to reduce the stress and strain in order to enjoy fully the purpose of the journey with this planned to be the product, rather than the process.

The use of television has caused considerable debate. How much more debate will be caused by the extended use of computers and other systems still to be designed. The development of an alert and open mind, flexible and adaptable to future needs must be encouraged in young children together with the firm foundation of basic skills and values.

TRAVELLING WITH YOUNG CHILDREN

It is usually a question of necessity rather than pleasure to travel with young children. They rarely appreciate the process once the novelty has worn off—probably a few minutes—and are impatient to conclude the experience. The physical restriction, usually necessary, together with boredom, are the aspects to be alleviated by a variety of strategies.

Babies normally travel well if they are warm, comfortable, satisfied of hunger and thirst and in a well-ventilated environment.

They often settle quickly to the sensation of movement and the noise of the engine. Those who attempt to make surroundings especially quiet for a baby may be in danger of reducing his or her confidence and security. The baby's most basic positive experience in the womb was rarely still for long and certainly far from silent.

Transport

PRAMS

There is such a wide variety of prams and pushchairs available now that it is chiefly a matter of personal preference once safety standards have been properly checked. Such vehicles need to fit in with the individual life style of the family, and the absence of the large coach built perambulator reflects the changes over the past decade or two.

Accepting that safety is ensured, it is vital to check the height of the handles. Many mothers spend hours of their lives in an uncomfortable and unhealthy position wheeling prams that are too low. Check also at regular intervals, that, if the pram is used for sleeping outside, there is sufficient room for the baby to stretch lengthwise.

CARRYING HARNESSES

There are many carrying harnesses on the market, some being better than others. Once again, it is a matter of personal preference and convenience but it is essential to try these articles before purchasing, using a child, if possible, or a burden of relative weight. It can be a feat of contortionist proportions to successfully harness oneself properly over outdoor clothing, in the absence of helping hands. Some of these contraptions are carried on the back, others in the front, and both have their market. Those babies carried in the front often appear to have their faces pressed in uncomfortable positions and seem to have a relatively boring view. Their necks are often unsupported when the child drops off to sleep. Those on the back appear to be adopting a more natural position and certainly have a commanding view of their environment when awake and travelling. A big advantage of harnesses is that children may accompany their parents inside stores and outside, on rambles where prams and pushchairs would be very difficult to negotiate. They are also much cheaper than prams, and babies are happy being close to the adult's body. Both harnesses and prams would seem to have their place in the life of today's children and adults.

Never discount the idea of buying a pram second-hand. Many have been used for a relatively short period and an overhaul and safety check will provide an adequate vehicle at a much lower capital cost.

WALKING

As children grow they will begin to appreciate the opportunity to walk themselves. To enjoy this experience in maximum safety, try to arrange such an activity whenever possible as part of a recreational outing. Other outings such as shopping or other purposeful journey are often limited in time, take concentration on the part of the adult, and result in frustration for both parties.

Remember, a small child may take three steps to one of the adult. A sad but familiar sight is one of a toddler, in order to stay with the adult, being obliged to keep up a trot. Appreciate that short legs tire in relation to the number of times they move backwards and forwards. Encourage the habit of walking for pleasure; it is an activity not favoured sufficiently by the young, due to the ease with which most of them are transported in early life. Later, however, it can provide one of the cheapest and most enjoyable ways in which to fill leisure time and maintain health, as well as learning at first hand about the natural environment.

It is relevant to mention that shoes *must* always be carefully chosen, fit well, and be suitable for their purpose. Shoes for walking should support in the correct places whilst leaving room for natural growth. The best that can be afforded should be purchased. Economize on other clothing in favour of footwear if necessary. Children will not suffer through wearing good second-hand clothes, but their feet may be permanently deformed leading to serious problems later in life through wearing ill-fitting shoes. It is not suffcient to ask the child if shoes are comfortable, as young complex bone formations will modify to the inappropriately shaped shoe.

It is often useful to carry a drink on moderately long excursions; individual children vary, but thirst is physically miserable and so easily remedied. Added to this the child will continue in a much happier frame of mind.

Take every opportunity to communicate basic road safety practice.

CARS

From the first few days of life, travel by car is experienced by many children and manufacturers of safety equipment have endeavoured to meet the needs of the young traveller. From harnesses for carrycots, to seats for the toddler and child, catering for the whole age range. Safely restrained children travel happily and adults can concentrate on the skills of driving.

Frequent stops are welcomed, both for refreshment and physical freedom. Try to choose a suitable turning, off the main highway, where children can run safely for a time. Lay-bys serve a very useful purpose but are noisy and potentially hazardous, both from the main stream of traffic and other users of the facility. It is beneficial for the driver to be able to relax away from the road.

Carry light refreshments: fluids such as cold milk or squash in warm weather; soup or warm milky drinks if it is cold. Biscuits will normally be sufficient unless the journey is very long. In any case avoid sticky or messy foods, as in the UK one can never guarantee the weather and picnics may have to take place in the car.

If the children are not good travellers offer a very light nongreasy meal before setting out, and stick to cool drinks, plain biscuits and boiled sweets on the journey. There are effective medications for prevention of travel sickness available from the chemist but many parents ease the situation by planning their journey to coincide with a familiar sleeping period, even travelling through the night.

Always carry something with which to wipe hands and face, even if only to refresh. A damp flannel sprinkled with a little eau de Cologne kept in a seal fresh container is useful. There are also prepared impregnated tissues sold in convenient dispensers.

According to the age of the children, make some simple plans for entertainment during the journey. 'I Spy' games are successful, as are taped stories or programmes. Magnetic or pegged board games appeal to a wide age range. Reading or knitting, involving constant attention with the head down, for some reason, seems to cause some people to feel nauseous, so is probably best discouraged. The intermittent attention required to fill in crosswords or puzzle books, presents few problems apart from the movement of the vehicle. Whatever is planned, try to avoid involving the driver. The high level of concentration and all-round alertness vital to safe driving on the fast motorways, is best allowed for by the absence of irrelevant intrusion.

Whether driving or travelling as a passenger, always make safety checks before setting out as well as following the recommended servicing programme: tyres including spares, oil, water, wipers, fluid for screen washer, first aid kit, jack, wheel brace, club memberships, are some basic check points. Other checks would cover the carrying of a warning triangle, an emergency windscreen, and spare petrol in an approved container. With long gaps between service stations, the latter is becoming more common.

TRAINS

Travelling by rail is fast and comfortable once you have actually boarded the train. The most tedious part is often the journey to the station, the waiting, and the difficulty in allowing for delays. It is an expensive way to travel, although there are often special offers which can considerably reduce this cost.

Refreshments are costly and difficult to collect from the distribution point, if there is no service in the carriage. It is advisable to take simple snacks and drinks, and dispense them in small quantities at regular intervals. There is nothing quite as successful as eating and drinking to relieve boredom. Once more, sleep is a welcome friend on long journeys.

Toileting children is often difficult both due to very limited space and the motion of the train; if the children are dressed simply the problem of organization in a confined space will be reduced. Carry the necessary articles to wipe hands and face.

Another consideration is that of the choice of packing cases. Remember that a child or children will need physical guidance. They may be too confused, distracted or simply pushed around by other travellers to be responsible for keeping near to those in charge of them. If heavy cases are mobile, using sets of wheels or casters, children can help to push them or hang on to them—at best the adult is better able to offer a spare hand. Most stations supply trolleys on which a very large burden of luggage can be transported very easily. The children can often ride comfortably at the same time.

AEROPLANES

Once again, it is usually after a journey that the real business of flying commences. Most countries are not served by sufficient airports to avoid some travellers having to cover considerable distances to reach one. Consequently, most adults will have to plan and consider more than one method of transport to reach destinations abroad. The initial method is likely to be one of those already covered, i.e. car or train.

Unfortunately for those with young children, travellers are requested to report to the air terminal well in advance of their time of departure. Add to this any delay and the happy anticipation can become sadly diluted. On the positive side, facilities at terminals are usually very good, special arrangements being available for babies and young children. The staff are helpful and well-informed.

In flight, children usually travel happily and the cabin staff are most attentive. If forwarned at the time of booking, they will arrange to carry any special foods and will certainly prepare any baby foods presented to them during the flight.

TELEVISION

The television is here to stay and, with few exceptions, children will have access to this appliance throughout their early years. Even if some parents choose not to have one, their friends will, as do many playgroups and early education establishments.

It is generally accepted that, used sensibly, television can inform, educate and entertain in a positive way. Indiscriminate use, however, as a pacifier, childminder or constant background, is detrimental to the optimum development of the child. Television is not a substitute in the child's world for the social and emotional nourishment provided by a caring adult. Although in many instances it has become so, it cannot replace social interaction at any age. It is a sophisticated tool of communication and should be used for the particular job, at the appropriate time.

Television can broaden the horizons of the human mind in a way that books and direct experience cannot, due to the limitations of such media. Even direct experience has its limitations, e.g. it is most unlikely that any young child, even when placed close to the natural habitat of a particularly nervous small animal, will get more than a fleeting glimpse of that animal. The child will, in fact, be lucky to get that. Through the medium of television access is gained to some of the most beautiful and sensitive wild-life films produced. Special effects speed up growth and movement, likewise they can slow such processes down. The extra information drawn from these films compared to what is naturally observed is amazing. Language is naturally extended and enriched, although it must be accepted that exposure to constant television transmission can just as easily extend language in an undesirable direction. Scenes of violence, criminal activities or moral decadence can sow the seeds of thought, where such ideas may otherwise never have been planted.

Early in life children should become accustomed to using television as a tool, with a valuable role to play in a technological age. A tool which should be switched off when not required, this being particularly difficult even for some adults to do.

Here are a few more arguments for inclusion of a television in the life of young children:

1 Current affairs are presented in a straightforward, generally unbiased way.

2 Distant places are brought to life.

3 Historical situations can be presented through drama, including social documentaries.

4 Programmes can be used as starting points if the group can commence with a common experience.

5 Adults without specific expertise can use the support of

presenters, communicating skills such as music, cookery, foreign languages or crafts.

Television has been blamed for increasing violence amongst the young people in the urban areas. Statistically, there is no real evidence either way, but it is illogical to presume that any single factor could be so responsible.

Video tapes

Video tape recorders are part of many children's lives and access to material is simple. Unscrupulous dealers have produced and circulated what are commonly termed 'video nasties'. There has been much publicity, but it would appear that the adults display a concern out of proportion with the reaction of many of the children. The children tend to regard the worst items as unrealistic and stupid, and seem unaffected by them. The problem really lies in the accessibility of the tapes to very young children and the danger of nervous or emotionally unstable children or adolescents being seriously disturbed.

Frequency of viewing

That television has killed the art of conversation may have some foundation, but within the pattern of human development, the possible effects will, hopefully, be short-lived. More realistically, it is probably the natural laziness in many which encourages the passive role adopted during long periods of viewing. What is disturbing is the record of hours spent by very young children in this passive role. This time would otherwise be spent largely in a communicative capacity, even if this relationship was with the environment, or self. It is the variety which nourishes the psyche and stimulates mental agility and growth.

The ability to be happy and contented in solitude perhaps is more likely to develop if early experience is broad and varied. Loneliness is different and is one of the saddest and most painful of all human experiences. Being alone is something which awaits many humans and some cope better than others. Television can play the role of companion up to a point, but everyone should be equipped psychologically to be happy alone, even for short periods. It seems to complete the being—'To be happy with oneself.'

Appendix 1
Basic Check Lists of Skills Required

Many skills are required within the day nursery to deal with the varying situations that arise when caring for children of different ages.

CARE OF CHILD

General care

Welcoming child in morning
Settling child with toys
Comforting unhappy child
Taking child to toilet
Changing a nappy
Washing or bathing a child
Nasal hygiene

Finger and toe nail care
Hair washing
Head inspection
Cleansing infested head
Potty training
Supervision of rest period

Health routine

Weighing and measuring
   routine

Ventilaton of play room

Care of sick child

General management
Taking temperature, pulse and
   respiration
Giving medication

Sponging child using tepid
   water
Providing toys

First aid
Application of:
   Bandages

Dressing

Practical care and treatment of:
Nappy rash
Cuts
Bruises
Nose bleeds
Child with temperature

Care of new child in nursery

Welcoming child into group
Introducing child to group
Involving child with activities
Comforting child when
distressed
Caring for child at rest time
Helping child to learn symbols
to identify personal property
Helping child to settle at
meal time
Building relationship with
parents

Caring for child with behavioural difficulties

Coping with a temper tantrum
Occupying an over-active child
Coping with an aggressive child
Encouraging a difficult eater

CARE OF BABY

Feeding

Milton method
Boiling utensils
Hygiene in milk room
Care of bottles and teats

PREPARATION OF MEALS

Dried milk feeds
Liquid milk feeds
Fruit juice
Liquidizing
Solid feeds

WEANING

Giving a baby:
Milk feeds
Tastes
Liquid tastes
Liquidized feeds
Solid feeds
Vitamin drops

General care

Holding a young baby
Cuddling a baby
Talking to a baby
Changing a nappy
Washing a baby
Bathing a baby
Providing stimulating toys
  for age ranges: 0-3, 3-6, 6-12
  and 12-18 months
Care of toys
Making pram

Making cot
Cleaning cot
Care of pots
Toilet training
General care and cleanliness of
  room
Care of flannel and towel
Treatment of cradle cap
Finger and toe care
Nasal hygiene

CREATIVE ACTIVITIES

Painting

Setting up and staffing
Easel painting
Wall painting

Mixing paints
Table painting
Floor painting

METHODS OF PAINTING

Finger
Foot
Bubble
String
Flick
Syringe
Car track

Doily
Spatula
Squeezy bottle
Ball
Texture
Straw
Butterfly

Printing

METHODS OF PRINTING

Block

Lego

Hand   Stickle-brick
Vegetable   Leaf
Cotton reel   Twig
Sponge

Collage

Presenting and staffing   Providing different textures

Junk modelling

Working with: Providing small domestic junk,
  Individual child   e.g. large boxes, tubes
  Small group

Dough

Staffing session   Mixing dough

Clay

Presenting and staffing   Care of clay—storing

Cooking

Measuring ingredients with   Preparing food for party
  children   with group
Baking sessions

Water play

Setting up and staffing:
  For toddlers in bath   For 3-year-olds in bath

Equipment:
  Pouring toys   In sink
  Floating and sinking   Washing dolls

Sieves

Capacity vessels

With bubbles

Washing dolls' clothes

Washing-up

Sand

Staffing play with small group   Sand: dry and wet

Table toys

Setting up and staffing:

Matching toys

Threading toys

Lotto

Simple board games

Colour games

Picture dominoes

Snap

Brick and block play with:

Individuals under 3 years

Small group under 3 years

Individuals 3-5 years

Small group 3-5 years

Presenting and stimulating play
with:

Lego

Stickle-brick

Matador

Multi-link cubes

Dolls' house

Garage

Farm yard

Zoo

Play people

Imaginative play

Providing and observing play in:

Wendy corner

Shop

Cave (table covered by blanket)

Dressing-up corner

Garden

Table displays

NATURE TABLES

Seed sowing and growing   Nature displays
Bean growing

INTEREST TABLE

Colour table   Conversation around interest
Texture table   table Leading conversations:
Shape table   Individual child
Seasonal table   Small group
Sound table

STORIES, BOOKS, RHYMES AND MUSIC

Story telling to a group

Without a book   With finger puppets
With a prop   With sound effects
With flannelgraph

Using books

Reading books: Reading a story book:
  With individual child   With individual child
  With small group   With small group

Poetry

Introducing a poem to a group   Provide activities to illustrate a
                                 poem, e.g. group pictures

Rhymes and finger play

Using finger rhymes with: Introducing new rhymes
  1-3 children   Singing rhymes with group
  A larger group

Sound games

Reminding children of familiar
sounds:
  Clock
  Wind
  Water

Make simple instruments with
  children
Listening skills

Movement with a group

Using a prop
Small group activity
Large group activity

Using some form of rhythm
and using music:
  With a small group
  With a large group

Using musical instruments

For children to listen
To accompany a group

Children using instruments to
  accompany a record or singing

Circle games

Supervising ring games, e.g. Little mousee, Sandy-boy.

PHYSICAL PLAY

Special care should be taken when setting-up and supervising physical and energetic play as accidents occur when children are running
around playing. Try to make the environment as safe as possible to
enable the children to play happily and safely.

Environment

Responsibility for outside play
  session
Setting-up climbing activities
with:
  Boxes
  Climbing frame

Bikes and tractors
Races
Ball play

Small group outings

Responsibility for taking small groups:

To the shops

For a walk

To the park

GENERAL CARE

Play equipment

Repair of books, dolls, toys

Care of book corner

Displaying child's work

Nursery Routine

Planning and equipping
nursery

Safety measures in building

Safety check of equipment

Safety check of toys

Planning week's menu

Cooking simple meals

Personal Hygiene

Cleanliness:

Hair

Nails

Skin

Clothing

Nursery Environment

Sweeping

Polishing

Damp-dusting

Disposal of refuse

Care of bathroom

Care of toilets

Children's clothes

Sewing on buttons   Marking flannels etc.
Minor repairs   Washing private clothes

MEETINGS AND SESSIONS TO BE ATTENDED

Doctor's visit   Review meeting
Setting room for doctor   Waiting list review
Attending immunization session   Social workers' team meeting
Speech therapist   Parents' meeting
Physiotherapist   Case conferences
Staff meetings   Child minder meeting
Allocation meeting

Appendix 2
Useful Addresses

Association for Spina Bifida and Hydrocephalus, Tavistock House North, Tavistock Square, London WC1H 9HJ, *Tel*: 01 388 1382

Asthma Research Council, 13 Pembridge Square, London W2 4EH, *Tel*: 01 229 1149

British Diabetic Association, 10 Queen Anne Street, London W1M 0BD, *Tel*: 01 323 1531

British Epilepsy Association, Crowthorne House, New Wokingham Road, Wokingham, Berkshire, *Tel*: 034 46 3122

British Rheumatism and Arthritis Association, 6 Grosvenor Crescent, London SW1X 7ER, *Tel*: 01 235 0902

Cancer Prevention Society, 102 Inveroran Drive, Glasgow, *Tel*: 041 942 6128

Childminders, 67 Marylebone High Street, London W1, *Tel*: 01 935 9763

Child Poverty Action Group, 1 Macklin Street, London WC2, *Tel*: 01 242 9149

Children's Aid Team, 662 High Road, London N17, *Tel*: 01 808 4965

Children's Book Centre Ltd., 229 Kensington High Street, London W8, *Tel*: 01 937 6314

Children's Music Theatre Ltd., 259 Harvist Road, London NW6, *Tel*: 01 960 8996

Children's Theatre (Polka), 240 The Broadway, London SW19, *Tel*: 01 543 4888

The Coeliac Society, PO Box 181, London NW2 2QY, *Tel*: 01 459 2440

Cystic Fibrosis Research Trust, 5 Blyth Road, Bromley, Kent BR1 3RS, *Tel*: 01 464 7211

Disabled Living Foundation, 346 Kensington High Street, London W14 8NS *Tel*: 01 602 2491

Dr Barnardo's, Tanner's Lane, Barkingside, Ilford, Essex, *Tel*: 01 550 8822

Foundation for the Study of Infant Deaths (Cot deaths), 23 St Peter's Square, London W6 9NW, *Tel*: 01 748 7768

The Haemophilia Society, PO Box 9, 16 Trinity Street, London SE1 1DE, *Tel*: 01 407 1010

Invalid Children's Aid Association, 126 Buckingham Palace Road, London SW1W 9BR, *Tel*: 01 730 9891

Leukaemia Research Fund, 43 Great Ormond Street, London WC1, *Tel*: 01 405 0101

Muscular Dystrophy Group of Great Britain, Natrass House, 35 Macaulay House, London SW4 0QP, *Tel*: 01 720 8055

National Association for Deaf/Blind and Rubella Handicapped Children, 311 Gray's Inn Road, London WC1, *Tel*: 01 278 1009

National Association for Gifted Children, 1 South Audely Street, London W1Y 6JS, *Tel*: 01 499 1188

National Association for Mental Health (MIND), 22 Harley Street, London W1N 2ED, *Tel*: 01 637 0741

National Association for the Welfare of Children in Hospital, Exton House, London SE1 8VE, *Tel*: 01 261 1738

National Childbirth Trust, 9 Queensborough Terrace, London W2 3TB, *Tel*: 01 221 3833

National Children's Bureau, 8 Wakley Street, London EC1, *Tel*: 01 278 9441

National Children's Home, 85 Highbury Park, London N5 1UD, *Tel*: 01 226 2033

National Council for One Parent Families, 255 Kentish Town Road, London NW5 2LX, *Tel*: 01 267 1361

National Deaf Children's Society, Charity Organisation, 45 Hereford Road, London W2, *Tel*: 01 229 9272

National Eczema Society, Tavistock House North, Tavistock Square, London WC1, *Tel*: 01 388 4097

National Society for Autistic Children, The Day Centre LtAP, 6 Florence Road, London W5, *Tel*: 01 579 6281

National Society for the Prevention of Cruelty to Children, 1 Riding House Street, London W1P 8AA, *Tel*: 01 580 8812

Parents Anonymous for Distressed Parents, 6 Manor Gardens, London N7, *Tel*: 01 263 5672/8918 (Lifeline)

Preschool Playgroups Association, Alford House, Aveline Street, London SE11 5DH, *Tel*: 01 582 8871

Royal National Institute for the Blind, 224 Great Portland Street, London W1N 6AA, *Tel*: 01 388 1266

Royal National Institute for the Deaf, 105 Gower Street, London WC1E 6AH, *Tel*: 01 387 8033

Safety in Playgrounds Action Group, 85 Dalston Drive, Didsbury, Manchester M20 0LQ

The Spastics Society, 12 Park Crescent, London W1N 4EQ, *Tel*: 01 636 5020

Bibliography

Ainsworth M. D. *et. al.* (1966) In Bowlby J. (ed.) *Maternal Care and Mental Health.* New York, Schocken.

Axline V. M. (1966) *Dibs: In Search of Self.* London, Gollancz.

Barth L. G. (1953) *Embryology.* New York, Holt, Rinehart & Winston.

Butterworth G. (1982) *Infancy and Epistomology. An Evaluation of Piaget's Theory.* London, St. Martin's Press.

Chase W. P. (1937) Colour Vision in Infants. *J. Exp. Psych.* 20, 203-22.

Copeland J. (1976) *For the Love of Ann.* London, Arrow.

Erickson E. (1967) *Childhood and Society.* London, Penguin.

Morris D. (1977) *Manwatching: Field Guide to Human Behaviour.* London, Cape.

Index